War on All Fronts

War on All Fronts

A Theory of Health Security Justice

Nicholas G. Evans

The MIT Press
Cambridge, Massachusetts
London, England

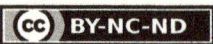
The MIT Press would like to thank the anonymous peer reviewers who provided comments on drafts of this book. The generous work of academic experts is essential for establishing the authority and quality of our publications. We acknowledge with gratitude the contributions of these otherwise uncredited readers.

This book was set in Stone Serif and Stone Sans by Westchester Publishing Services. Printed and bound in the United States of America.

Library of Congress Cataloging-in-Publication Data

Names: Evans, Nicholas G., 1985– author.
Title: War on all fronts : a theory of health security justice / Nicholas
    G. Evans.
Description: Cambridge, Massachusetts : The MIT Press, [2023] | Includes
    bibliographical references and index.
Identifiers: LCCN 2022029551 | ISBN 9780262545433 (paperback) |
    ISBN 9780262374217 (epub) | ISBN 9780262374224 (pdf)
Subjects: MESH: Communicable Disease Control | Disease Outbreaks—
    prevention & control | Public Health—ethics | Security Measures—
    ethics | Social Justice—ethics | Health Policy | Politics
Classification: LCC RA643 | NLM WA 110 | DDC 362.1969—dc23/eng/20221110
LC record available at https://lccn.loc.gov/2022029551

10 9 8 7 6 5 4 3 2 1

In memory of Shi De Chuan, who taught me about war

Contents

A Note on Acronyms   ix

Acknowledgments   xi

1 Introduction   1
2 The War Metaphor   19
3 Reconciling Military and Public Health Ethics   37
4 The Impersonal Account of Disease   63
5 The Moral Foundations of the Public Health State   91
6 Justly Declaring an Emergency   115
7 The Ethics of Liberty-Limiting Measures   133
8 Drawing up the Troops: Waging War on Disease   153
9 Peace in Public Health   167
10 Whose War? Policy and Public Health Politics   177
    Epilogue: Emergency Innovation   189

Notes   205
Index   257

A Note on Acronyms

In general, acronyms make life harder for books that aim to cross disciplines. Here, I will use only a few. I will refer to the disease colloquially known as "COVID" as COVID-19, reflecting its World Health Organization designation as "coronavirus disease 2019." In early chapters, or when referencing early work prior to this naming convention, I will refer to "nCoV-2019," or "novel coronavirus 2019." The virus that causes this disease is called "SARS-CoV-2" or "severe acute respiratory disease coronavirus 2."

In referring to international agencies and conventions, I will use their standard English acronyms: UN for United Nations, WHO for World Health Organization, and so on. WHO generally has no definite article; that is, it is WHO, whereas "The Who" is a band. WHO oversees the International Health Regulations (IHR), within which there is an instrument described as a Public Health Emergency of International Concern (PHEIC). The Who performed "Baba O'Reilly," which is a great song, and two years younger than the IHR; it is three years older than the Biological and Toxin Weapons Convention (BTWC).

I will occasionally refer to policy or executive agencies in various countries: the US Centers for Disease Control (US CDC), Department of Defense (US DOD), the United Kingdom Health Security Executive (UK HSE), and so on. I typically add the country first to any acronym, as many regions have the same names for similar bodies. There is a US CDC, but there is also a Nigerian CDC; within the United States, there is also, for example, a CDC for the state of Maine.

In general, all other names will not be subject to acronyms. My apologies to anyone for whom this practice strikes as inconvenient. One thing I have learned while working *in* health security, however, is that as a field that crosses disciplines, you can easily get lost if you are a public health person, for example, listening to the national security people talk. The converse is the same, though admittedly my colleagues at US DOD tend to be the worst offenders, and US federal employees in general need to quit acronyms. It is my hope that the smattering I provide obviates the need for them to go cold turkey.

Acknowledgments

This book was commissioned, drafted, and written in 2020, revised in 2021, and edited in 2022. It contains, however, research of approximately eight years. Many people aided in its development, though all errors remain solely my responsibility.

First thanks go to my editor, Phillip Laughlin, and the staff at the MIT Press. Without Phil's enthusiasm for me, and the project, I wouldn't be where I am now.

Next, to my wife Kelly Hills, for providing considerable feedback and conversation about some of the ideas within this work, her work as coauthor on a number of ethics and infectious disease papers cited in this book, tolerating my decision to do a *second* book in 2020 as I was finishing my first, and entertaining our cats at times when they were being needy (which is always, bless them).

Next, to the broad array of individuals whose comments on drafts of chapters, and at talks on which sections have been based, have helped this project develop. Special thanks go to Matthew Watson, Tom Inglesby, and Jaime Yassif for comments at the Johns Hopkins Center for Health Security's Emerging Leaders in Biosecurity Initiative Research Symposium in 2017. Additional thanks go to Paul Kelleher, Debra Matthews, Efthimios Parasidis, Glenn Cohen, Chris Park, Christine Grady, Danielle Wenner, Mara Buchbinder, Govind Persad, Matthew Peterson, Brent Kious, Maria Merritt, Lorenzo Servitje, Amanda Moodie, Yong-Bee Lim, and Jennifer Blumenthal-Barby for their helpful feedback on earlier drafts of this work in whole or part. Many thanks to the spring 2022 Planetary Law class at Georgetown University for their discussion of chapters 4 and 5. And my appreciation to the attendees of the Edgewood annual talk series in Andover, Massachusetts, and to Toby Hoades and Bill Campbell, in particular, for their comments on my work.

Putting this work together required working in a number of disparate policy worlds. Here, I am particularly indebted to Emily Ricotta, who provided advice on how epidemiological features of infectious disease might change my conclusions. She is one of only a few people to talk through the entire book with me more than once. Emily Kelley and Mary Lancaster provided insight into how my arguments might look from the perspective of defense experts. And Anna Muldoon's combination of on-the-ground public health experience, biodefense policy, and humanities scholarship was invaluable and finds expression in every chapter. Many thanks to Colin Carlson for humoring me with questions and ecology respectively, and not freaking out when I subsequently binged his body of work over a few days.

Many thanks to my collaborators on the various COVID-19 projects in which I took part, who aren't already mentioned elsewhere: Zack Beger, Ross Silverman, Brianna Smith, Jennifer Kwan, Julia Lynch, Erin Ice, Denna Costa, Blake Hereth, Ashton Sorrels, Paul Tubig, Hannah Davis, and Rocco Casagrande.

This wouldn't have been possible without the support of friends, and I am particularly indebted to my fellow Australian expatriate and health security colleague Alexandra Phelan, who kept me company—and kept my understanding of global health law honest. Thank you for your support through the lonely pandemic years we've been through already, and I hope I can provide the same in the years to come. Here's to a bike ride, a decent cup of coffee, and a crumpet with Vegemite one day.

My thanks to my dean, Luis Falcón, and department chair, John Kaag, for helping me through my tenure application the year I wrote the first version of this manuscript. Thanks to Provost Joseph Hartman, and Chancellor Jacqueline Maloney, for the endorsement that resulted in my successful promotion with tenure to associate professor.

This work was possible thanks to the generous funding of the National Science Foundation (#1734521), Greenwall Foundation Faculty Scholars Program, Davis Educational Foundation, and US Air Force Office of Scientific Research (#FA9550-21-1-0142 P0002), whose combined support provided the material basis for some of this research, and the salary support that gives me time to write. Thanks to my program officers and directors on these projects: Fred Kronz, Michelle Groman, Leanne Greeley Bond, and Laura Steckman.

Finally, to the aforementioned cats: Harley (RIP), Lexi, and Inky.

1 Introduction

This is a book about war. Imagined, metaphorical war, but one with a catastrophic toll all the same. It is a book about what it means to be at war, to do battle, and on what terms we win and lose.

The "war" I have in mind is the war against communicable disease. This war is metaphorical because literal wars are wars between humans. But efforts to respond to infectious diseases have for at least the last thirty years become increasingly *securitized*, conceived of in terms of national and global security. This has led to the formation of the field of "health security," which is the subject of this book.[1]

As a metaphor, drawing a comparison between war and infectious disease is a form of analogy. And in places, this analogy seems to bear significant weight. Public health crises, and especially those caused by disease pandemics, may require mobilization of extensive resources in response. They may require us to make hard decisions about resource constraints even when we are prepared, and equally hard decisions about preparation during times of relative peace. And they may inform the structure of our most basic social institutions in the service of protecting individuals and communities from catastrophe. Armed conflict is a social, political, and ethical issue on a grand scale; so too is the war against communicable disease.

Rather than simply claim a mere analogy, however, in this work I claim that there is a relationship between the principles that govern the ethics of armed conflict, and those that should govern our responses to public health crises. I call this a theory of *just health security*, itself a reference to the tradition of just war theory that has dominated the ethics of war for a millennium. As a work of philosophy, my aim is to show how an understanding of the ethics of armed conflict provides a defensible view of a just, securitized public health ethics. As a work of health security, my aim is to formulate an account to guide action, particularly as the world deals with the fallout from the coronavirus disease 2019 (COVID-19) pandemic.

The War on COVID-19

This book is not about COVID-19, but it is inspired by the respiratory illness caused by severe acute respiratory syndrome coronavirus 2 (SARS-CoV-2). COVID-19 emerged on December 31, 2019, with a report of a cluster of pneumonia cases of unknown etiology in Wuhan, capital of Hubei province in the People's Republic of China (PRC).[2] By January 21, 2020, when the World Health Organization (WHO) began its first situation report on what was then called "novel coronavirus 2019 (nCoV-2019)," 282 cases had been reported, of which all but four had been in China, and all were connected to Wuhan.[3] Already, warnings had been issued about the possibility of exponential growth in cases, with some focusing on the Lunar New Year celebration in China scheduled for January 25 as a source of mass movement through the nation, and thus movement of individuals infected but not yet ill with the virus.[4]

Those warnings were justified. By January 31, 2020, WHO confirmed 9,826 cases globally.[5] The day before, WHO Director General Tedros Adhanom Ghebreyesus declared the virus a public health emergency of international concern (PHEIC);[6] a day later, Massachusetts would report its first case as a college student returned to Boston from Wuhan.[7] By then, 132 cases had been recorded as travel from China pushed the virus into twenty-three countries.[8] The pattern would repeat, doubling once every ten days or so.

Public fears mounted, but with the exception of proactive and prepared nations such as the Republic of Korea, whose experience with Middle Eastern respiratory syndrome had led to reforms in its public health infrastructure,[9] most countries did nothing. It would not be until March that new hotspots would raise alarms: in Italy, of physicians increasingly driven to ration ventilator support for critical cases,[10] and in Iran, where the press would report breathlessly of "burial pits in Iran so vast that they're visible from space."[11] But by that time, it was too late.

Cancel Everything

Most developed nations finally responded to the threat of COVID-19 in March. Responses were varied. Travel restrictions were imposed not just externally, but within local jurisdictions. Stay-at-home orders were applied and enforced, some nations locked their populations down with police enforcement, in-person schooling was canceled, and nonessential businesses and restaurants were closed. Contact tracing systems were used to try and place individuals in the context of transmission events and locate other cases. Most nations did some of these; a rare few did all of them. Some did none.

The media landscape, and health messaging within it, was a maelstrom. Some authors referred to "flattening the curve"—that is, the epidemic curve of daily cases that dictated when resource limits would be exceeded in hospitals and public health agencies. Still others referred to variations on "the hammer and the dance," referring to sequential implementation of restrictions and reopening to suppress the virus until a vaccine could be produced.[12] Commentators leaned into the "Swiss cheese" model for risk reduction in which layers of risk mitigation policies protect a population through their sum: one group, in what must be a self-defeating attempt to improve public communications, attempted to rename this the "Emmentaler cheese" model.[13] Into this morass—fueled by chaotic messaging from Donald J. Trump, the forty-fifth president of the United States, who among other things likened his political opponents' concerns over COVID-19 to a hoax[14]—stepped a slew of other messages. Some of those messages were well meaning, others were pernicious and exploitative.

Often scarcer than ICU beds, or respirators, was the political will to act, and continue to act, to suppress and eliminate the virus. In his article "Cancel Everything," political scientist Yasha Mounk made the following case for extensive suppression tactics to deal with COVID-19:

1. cases of COVID-19 were increasing in an exponential fashion (i.e., a person infected with the virus would on average infect more than one other person);
2. COVID-19 had a higher fatality rate than seasonal influenza, and thus constituted a grave threat;
3. only "extreme social distancing"—according to Mounk, canceling public gatherings, so-called self-quarantine, and sealing off Wuhan and the province of Hubei—would curtail the spread of the virus.[15]

From this, Mounk concluded that social distancing was not only permissible; "serious forms of social distancing" were necessary.

What best defined the political moment were two corollaries made by Mounk. The first corollary was, given social distancing would be ineffective if people could not get treatment or afford to stay home from work, that the government needed to enact additional policies. He argued that the government should take on the costs of medical treatment, grant paid sick leave to stricken workers, promise not to deport undocumented workers who seek medical help, and invest in rapid expansion of ICU facilities. But second, Mounk claimed the federal government would not enact the above, and thus it was up to *individuals* to pursue social distancing.

The measures that eventuated were certainly not sufficient. Indeed, it is hard to find a single government worldwide whose track record would be unassailable over the course of the pandemic. But the transference of responsibility to individuals, and Mounk's insistence on measures such as broad travel restrictions *without* social support, which cut against the ethical and scientific standards of public health, would become a disaster in its own right.[16] Mounk was not alone, and governments and popular messaging articulated "flatten the curve" as an individual strategy but never came up with an adequate plan of what to do next.[17] By the end of 2021, two years into the pandemic, even countries that began with excellent records of preventing the transmission of the virus would start to collapse, as variant after variant of SARS-CoV-2—the "delta" and "omicron" variants in particular— would overrun health systems and regions that had lapsed in their vigilance, leading to case counts and deaths higher than the first waves of the pandemic and the return of overflowing ICUs and crisis standards of care.

The Long War (on Everything)

Amidst all of this, war was declared on COVID-19. One of the earliest references to this war came from the PRC during its early reckoning with COVID-19, when Ma Guoqiang, Chinese Communist Party secretary for Wuhan, described the increased response to then-named nCoV-2019:

> Wuhan must strictly implement the public health emergency action level-II requirements set by Hubei province, completely enter a state of war and put resolute efforts to curb the spread of the novel coronavirus.[18]

The same week, the *Wall Street Journal* described the shaky footing of global pandemic preparedness efforts in military terms, noting that efforts by China to exclude Taiwan from the WHO hampered the "war on epidemics."[19] President Trump would follow suit when America finally began its belated response, declaring himself a "wartime president" against an invisible enemy. He used the rhetoric to advance a narrative of self-sacrifice, invoking the costs of World War II and claiming "We must sacrifice together, because we are all in this together, and we will come through together. It's the invisible enemy. That's always the toughest enemy, the invisible enemy."[20]

The war metaphor would be used to advocate for strategies used against the outbreak; to describe the "front lines" where healthcare workers[21]—but curiously, not "essential workers" such as grocery store clerks—battled the virus. It would be used in more literal senses, such as invoking the US Defense Production Act, a piece of legislation authorizing the government to commandeer industry and other resources in aid of national defense.[22] Still more would use it to describe the virus's "rampage through the body."[23] It would be used supportively to promote ideas about the outbreak, but also critically to distinguish failures in "strategy" and "tactics" in pandemic response. And it would be used to describe the dead as they overflowed hospital morgues into makeshift tents in communities.[24]

This is hardly a new phenomenon, and Americans are perhaps the best known for their zeal at declaring war on everything from nations to abstract concepts, having long perfected the art of war metaphors. President Nixon declared "war on cancer" in 1971 with the signing of the National Cancer Act, mobilizing the National Cancer Institute and creating the National Cancer Advisory Board.[25] This war has continued through the twenty-first century, incorporating parallel metaphors such as the "cancer moonshot"—which, for those familiar with the history of the space race, know is just as militant.[26] We have had wars on HIV/AIDS, on the SARS-CoV-1 virus that spread through the world in 2002–2003, on Ebola virus disease, and even on antimicrobial resistance[27]—each disease with different etiologies and mechanisms of action, prevalence levels, morbidity and mortality, treatment pathways, and public health status. The instinct to use war as a metaphor is hardly unique to the United States, however, and is a rallying cry to mobilize resources and draw attention.[28] But over the last forty years it has become increasingly central to the calculus of public health as the emergence of the term "health security" situating public health—and responding to communicable disease in particular—as a national security concern.

And, like most metaphorical wars, the world lost the war against COVID-19.

The War within the War

It may seem premature to declare the war on COVID-19 lost, but the span of two years bears this out. Five million people had died by the beginning of 2022.[29] Economies in ruins: at its worst in April 2020, 14 percent of workers in the United States—1 in 7 Americans—were unemployed, and half of those still unemployed a year later;[30] worldwide, almost 9 percent of the world's population was out of work.[31] Other diseases were neglected and left to run rampant, such as a "comeback" for tuberculosis in Peru.[32] A terrifying increase in domestic violence occurred worldwide, leading *Time* magazine to refer to it as a "pandemic within the pandemic."[33] Plus an educational crisis,[34] and more. And more cases daily by the end of 2021, as in the worst of the first wave. By 2022, much of the world had stopped counting the toll with any precision, except insofar as excess mortality from COVID-19 remained high.

These losses, moreover, are not equally distributed—just as in war. Of those unemployed in the United States as a result of the early pandemic, the majority were service workers, who experienced an unemployment rate of 40 percent at the peak of the crisis,[35] affecting predominantly people of color, women, young, and people with disabilities.[36] In the United Kingdom, more than 50 percent of COVID deaths were among people with disabilities.[37] And the long-term sequelae of COVID-19, the "Long COVID" as it is known, will potentially leave millions with lingering illness.[38] As New Zealand, one of the staunchest opponents of the virus, announced relaxing its pandemic lockdown standards, it was predicted that indigenous Māori are more likely to suffer as a result than white Kiwis.[39]

The obvious response—and one made by a reviewer of this book—is that the early arrival of vaccines signaled a profound victory over the virus. It is true vaccines exist, but the where and for whom of vaccination highlight the depths of the failure to wage war on COVID. Fifteen percent of the world's population possesses 60 percent of the world's vaccination supply, and by the end of 2021 only 2 percent of people in low-income countries had received one dose of a COVID-19 vaccine, compared to 65 percent of people in high-income countries.[40] All the while, rich countries continue to hoard vaccines for additional boosters as new variants of SARS-CoV-2 challenge their population.[41] While high-income countries vaccinated at a high rate compared to their poorer neighbors, their initial successes were coupled with a premature easing of so-called social distancing measures, and new spikes in cases. Many experts and policymakers, it seems, became comfortable with the SARS-CoV-2 virus circulating in the developed world in the medium to long term so long as it didn't result in hospitalization or death for the vaccinated, and so long as the economy remained stable enough. For the rest of the world political will has faded, and needless deaths have accrued.

This is not D-Day or Iwo Jima. This is at best a public health Afghanistan. It is more likely the infectious disease equivalent of the Charge of the Light Brigade, a health security Gallipoli, or even a public health Stalingrad. This is not a war of heroes. It is an unending slog.

Individuals who have securitized healthcare are thus struck with a problem: declaring war on COVID, as with other things that aren't actually war, does not actually lead to successful—much less just—outcomes. If anything, it is associated with failure more than success. This book, at a fundamental level, is about addressing whether there is a just way to wage war on infectious disease.

Health Security

At the heart of the war on COVID-19—or Ebola, or AIDS, or antimicrobial resistance, or some future "Disease X"—is the idea of health security. Health security is less a discipline united by a common set of epistemic norms and methodologies and more a cross- and interdisciplinary collection of activities centered around the idea of health and public health as a component of national security. Lorna Weir has documented the rise of the concept of "(global) health security" as an act of securitization beginning in the 1990s, with Canadian and US efforts to define and then incorporate into global governance the concept of "emerging infectious diseases," and then "render WHO responsible for preventing the international transmission of emerging infectious diseases."[42] Through the early 2000s, this became a task to which WHO, driven by what Weir identifies as the interests of the Global North, responded by outlining a system of disease surveillance and control they termed the "world on alert," a metaphor explicitly tying health to security. It ultimately dovetailed with ongoing efforts to update the international health regulations (IHR) and after the terrorist attacks of September 2001, became explicitly associated with responding to chemical, biological, radiological, and nuclear attacks. These two factors, among others, led to proposed IHR drafts that explicitly favored a "threat-defense" conception of public health, and one that focused not on responding to endemic diseases but to emerging diseases that crossed international borders. The use of the language of threat, in particular, Weir rightly identifies as the language of security rather than public health conceptions of risk.[43]

In 2022 WHO defines "health security," or rather "global public health security," as activities required, both proactive and reactive, to minimize the danger and impact of acute public health events that endanger people's health across geographical regions and international boundaries.[44] Two central preoccupations emerge from this definition's historical antecedents. The first is an (albeit not exclusive) concern with infectious disease, and in particular disease pandemics caused either by natural events or biological weapons. The second is the framing of these events as a threat to national and global communities, and the continuation of the social fabric and international order.

When it comes to bioterrorism, health security arguably arises from concerns of developed nations about state and nonstate biological weapons activity,[45] and the risk of a deliberate or accidental release of a biological agent into the human population.[46] This focus predates the twenty-first century[47] but received considerably more interest at the turn of the millennium following the anthrax attacks of 2001 and the emergence of "dual-use research" that could be used to advance both the beneficial and malicious uses of the life sciences.[48]

Next, health security deals with conventional public health issues by recognizing naturally arising pathogens as a national security threat in their own right. While there are many ways to discuss this, there is perhaps none more extreme—or indicative—than the claim made in an editorial in *Nature* during the SARS epidemic that "nature is the ultimate bioterrorist." This claim was followed with the purported good news that "the genome sequence of the prime suspect . . . will become available any day now. This should help to reveal where the virus came from, suggest reasons for its lethality, and speed the development of rapid tests for its presence."[49] The conception of nature as a perceived threat predates SARS. Threats imply an intentionality, an obviously nonsensical concept in the case of the virus itself.[50] But they also imply a right to self-defense which, famously, does not require intention to be justified.

The idea of self-defense is critical to American conceptions of public health in general. The landmark case in public health, *Jacobson v. Massachusetts*, upheld the authority of states to enforce compulsory vaccination laws. In that ruling, the court held that:

> Upon these principles of self-defense, or paramount necessity, a community has the right to protect itself against an epidemic of disease which threatens the safety of its members.

Jacobson will become important in later chapters, in part because it defines a quintessentially American interpretation of public health in the context of disease epidemics. That interpretation holds that infectious *people* present a threat to their community, against which the community has a right to self-defense. Interestingly, it also invokes the principle of necessity, which brings up a longer and older tradition of jurisprudence that covers state responses not only to particular exigent circumstances but also to individual rights and responses in the face of the overriding demands of nature.[51] Under *Jacobson* a community is justified in exercising power, even coercive or violent power, against others in order to protect against the "threat" of infectious disease.

Not all concepts of health security stem from analogy to personal self-defense but may touch on other elements of security. While Australia has a *National Health Security Act*, much of its public health powers mobilized against pandemic disease are through its *Biosecurity Act* of 2015. This, however, is a replacement not for a human security instrument, but an initially *agricultural* instrument, the *Quarantine Act* of 1908. This act was first designed to provide the federal government of Australia with powers over quarantine against infectious diseases that superseded those of the states but was over time amended to encompass a wide range of human and animal pathogens.

The relationship between human and animal security dovetails with the trend toward health security as a war in response to the threat of nature itself. This has manifested in the emergence, for example, of climate change as a health security issue.[52] The 2018 Zika virus outbreak brought with it the fear that as climate changes, and host ranges of mosquitoes expand, the likelihood that Zika and other *Aedes Aegypti*-borne diseases will infect Americans will increase.[53] Since the elimination of yellow fever in the US, few mosquito-borne illnesses have established themselves on the continent. With that potential change has come increased pressure to deploy novel methods such as gene drives, and genetically modified mosquitos to eliminate the creature the Centers for Disease Control (CDC) refers to as the "World's Deadliest Animal."[54]

Public Health Ethics and Health Security

Public health ethics became entwined with health security following the anthrax attacks of fall 2001 in the US. One central issue that concerned both was the possibility that an adversary of the US would be in a position to attack using a biological weapon, requiring the allocation of extreme amounts of human and medical resources to counter. The number of deaths involved depends on the course of action but estimates of a particularly successful attack with a sophisticated anthrax weapon were believed to be in the tens to hundreds of thousands.[55]

What emerged in the wake of this was the development of both legal and ethical frameworks to address exigent circumstances such as bioterrorism, a literature bolstered first by the emergence of SARS in 2003, highly pathogenic avian influenza H5N1 in 2005, and the IHR reforms that followed.[56]

A central concern for authors, and one this book takes up, is what to do in extreme public health crises where human rights conflict with broader utilitarian concerns around saving lives. To this end, a popular framework for public health ethical decision-making was developed, describing a system of tradeoffs that recognize common moral commitments, and a framework for deciding when individual interests could be overridden in the pursuit of public health priorities.[57] It claimed that individual interests were overridable just in case a public health action was effective, necessary, had risks proportionate to its benefits, was the least infringing measure available, and publicly justifiable.

This framework, which I describe in full in chapter 3, is also significant in that its author list includes the architect of the US Model State Health Emergency Powers Act (MSHEPA), which was ultimately used by states within the US to enact legislation that governs emergency responses to bioterrorism or other public health disasters.[58] This model act became one of the earliest instantiations of modern health security, and its ultimate use in state legislation would become the basis for political action against COVID-19, for better or worse.

However, the concern about mass casualty events such as bioterrorism and pandemics, and the theme that emerged within that literature that individual rights could and should be overridden in the name of public health, has not been without its critics. As soon as the framework and its subsequent instantiation in policy appeared, critics remarked that leaning into a policy that countenanced rights infringement would undo the hard work of activists and scholars, particularly in the context of HIV/AIDS, to center human rights in health. Accompanying this were concerns about the internal consistency of the principles described in the framework, to what extent they could guide action, and how the presumption of certain values underpinning them would translate outside of the American-centric author group and context in which the framework arose.

Having read this framework in graduate school, where I was also writing on military ethics, one of the things that struck me about the principles is how closely they hewed to the tradition of just war theory, which (at least in its orthodox formulation) contains a set of principles governing when it is morally permissible to declare war, and how one should wage war. This book makes the case that this connection is not an accident—historically or philosophically. But its interpretation misses some critical features that the ethics of war can provide us. More importantly, the ethics of war gives us a way to think constructively about the value of rights in public health, and what it means to protect the people who hold them from, and during, emergencies.

Methods, Limits, and Structure of This Book

This book provides a novel theory of *just health security* and its relation to the practice of conventional public health (and public health ethics). Methodologically, I draw on the literature from armed conflict, with which public health ethics—or public health ethics that considers security—shares common principles, but which sometimes lack a set of deeper normative commitments. I argue that like just war theory, as a view that begins at pacifism and then steps back to ask under what limited conditions it is ever permissible to kill, so too should just health security begin with the idea that public health at its heart should hold human rights as critical, only in the most extreme of circumstances allowing those rights to be infringed upon, and doing so with an aim to quickly and justly restore a community after an emergency.

This is a preliminary work in some respects and is inspired by two works, neither of which are in public health. First, I draw strongly from Larry May's *Contingent Pacifism*. Like May in that book, my intention is to provide an argument that people will take seriously. It is not my intention to provide an airtight version of this novel theory, and indeed it will become clear that much more work may need to be done in order for that to arise. Rather, it is my intention that this argument is one that the reader—even if not persuaded by it in whole or even in part—will take to be a serious contender for a moral basis of health security. Indeed, while normally reserved for the acknowledgements section, I am indebted to Larry for a number of conversations more than thirteen years ago at the Australian National University about the ethics of war, conversations that have stuck with me and inform the larger project here.

My second aim is to provide an account of something with which people are familiar—or at least, a wide segment of people in the health sciences and humanities—but is increasingly subject to a series of argumentative moves that contain misleading or even bad faith arguments that shield particular visions of public health and national security from reasonable critique. In this aim, I am indebted to Hugh LaFollette's *A Defense of Gun Control*. LaFollette, born and raised in Louisiana and a longtime gun owner and hunter, mounts an argument in that book that he acknowledges himself is one he has taken time to arrive at: that gun control in the United States is not only morally required, but able to be implemented in a way that accounts for good faith defenses of the right to possess firearms. The argument LaFollette constructs, however, is one that deeply considers what is required for a defense of guns, or gun control, to be in good faith to begin with. In the same way, rather than either uncritically accepting the tenets of health security or rejecting the move to securitized health out of hand, I wish to provide a reconstruction of health security in terms that are defensible and compelling, before I describe its implications and limits.

These two inspirations come together to provide an account of health security that on the one hand is grounded in a theory of national and global security, acknowledging that even legitimate visions of national and global security entail state coercion; but on the other hand, the moral content of that vision should commit us to surprising, and indeed peaceful conceptions of state and human rights. Even if we believe coercive public health practices are justified in the name of national security, May's work provides a thoroughgoing analysis we can apply to states that consistently fail to meet the standard required of them in the real world, and what we should do with knowledge of their failures. LaFollette provides the means to rebuild an account of public health that is aligned with the best insights into the metaphor that public health is national security, before applying an analysis that takes seriously the demands of justice.

Throughout this book, I use the phrase "communicable disease." While the main examples I use are infectious diseases, and the US CDC regards communicable diseases as interchangeable with infectious diseases, I want to caution against this restrictive view. Some disease "epidemics" have a communicable nature, but that communicability is arguably totally social in nature. The most common of these I will refer to is the overdose epidemic gripping North America, passed through communities, between generations, and across regions. But there may be others: depression is communicable as a "social contagion," for example, and environmental disasters may have long-standing and even intergenerational effects or have reservoirs that continue to "spread" the disease beyond a single point of exposure. Many of the claims in this book are applicable to this wider set of communicable diseases, and the application of health security to attempt to solve things like overdoses. My account provides a guide to why and how, from a political-philosophical standpoint, treating "diseases of poverty" with the same tools as respiratory diseases is *possible*, but requires radically rethinking both.

Many of the examples I use are located in the US, though not all. One reviewer has suggested to me that I make this book entirely about health security in the US. I don't want to pretend that my position as an Australian living and working in the US is irrelevant to my perspective and analysis. Certainly the trauma of living through the US response to COVID-19—and with an immunocompromised spouse—has been a huge impact on this book. But my claims about the nature of public health threats do not depend on the passport held by the person vulnerable to those threats. And the arguments in chapter 5, in particular, depend on the nation-state, but not its particular American instantiation. The illustrations are US focused, but the analysis should be applicable, perhaps with additional twists, to many if not most other nations.

In the next chapter, I subject the war metaphor to detailed analysis. Starting with COVID-19, I provide examples to sketch what it means for public health, and in particular infectious disease, to pose a threat to the security of individuals and communities that lends itself to the war metaphor: threat, mobilization of resources, high stakes decision-making, and the role of social institutions in security. I then turn to the primary critique of the war metaphor, grounded in securitization theory. This theory claims that, at best, the war metaphor inadvertently places an existential finger on priority setting in health, and at worst is a mere performance that serves vested interests. I ultimately reject this critique of securitization, or at least its normative instantiation. I argue instead that the critique shows why the war metaphor, and its instantiation in public health norms and policies, needs to be deeply examined in the context of ethical and political-philosophical theories about state power.

What follows in chapter 3 connects the war metaphor to public health. The most obvious way, I argue, is through the orthodox view of public health ethics. I articulate this view in detail and describe how it tracks important elements of the war metaphor. The debate between critics and supporters of this partly securitized version of public health ethics is instructive in understanding the war metaphor in ethical and political-philosophical terms. I argue that the most compelling argument for securitized public health ethics is the strong connection between the orthodox view and just war theory, the millennia-old theory of the justification for going to and killing in war. I show how this connection manifests and determines that a first step in a theory of just health security, or securitized public health, is justifying public health as appropriately the function of a nation-state.

Establishing this justification is the focus of chapter 4. I argue for an *impersonal account of disease* as the appropriate target of public health institutions, in which the appropriate "enemy" is the causative agent of disease itself, but not the victim of that disease. I compare this account to theories of noncombatant immunity in military ethics and show how both accounts provide a view to (a) the appropriate risks innocent people may be exposed to in responding to a threat, (b) the kinds of liability the state and its proxies must assume for the purpose of responding to a public health threat, and (c) our obligations to avoid the material conditions that lead to public health emergencies.

Chapter 5 then focuses on the appropriate institutional home for public health. Beginning with a reflection on the degree to which federalism has largely undermined the response effort to COVID-19 in the US, I argue that a critical step in health security is to establish public health not as a function of government *simpliciter*, but of the highest authoritative form of governance available to us—in this case, the nation-state. I then examine three broad political-philosophical theories: libertarianism, liberal contract theories (with a focus on the work of John Rawls), and utilitarianism. After discussing their limits and earlier attempts at plural theories of public health ethics, I argue a central problem in justifying a robust public health state is a *deep pluralism* around what kinds of values are important. I then turn to Michael Moehler's recent contractarian account of a minimal moral state and show how even this account of political philosophy from pure instrumental reason can provide a justification for a robust public health state, albeit one that at times must override individual rights or interests in the service of collective welfare. I sketch some limits of this account to return to at the end of the book: in particular, questions about legitimacy, authority, and assurance in contemporary states.

Chapter 6 concerns the declaration of public health emergency. Starting at the declaration of COVID-19 as a PHEIC and working backward, I argue that a central gap in public health ethics is a lack of systematic treatment of public health emergencies as distinct phenomena from "public health peace." I show why this gap explains some of the justified critiques from chapter 3 against the orthodox view and then offer a framework for declaring a public health emergency ethically. This framework explains why we ought not to use forced quarantine or other measures in nonemergent but serious public health events such as bad flu seasons, and thus generate a normative regime that can successfully conceive of rights-respecting public health during "peacetime," while accommodating rare emergency cases in which rights might be justifiably infringed upon for community safety. I then expand on the previous chapter's account of necessity and last resort as a component of this declaration framework as informing duties of states prior to emergencies. I turn finally to an obvious objection—that this framework unduly constrains public health practice—and examine it through the lens of the military ethics debates around the use of force short of war, and of supreme emergency.

Chapter 7 addresses the classic public health ethics issue of the use of "liberty limiting measures" including surveillance, measures that increase social distance, mandatory vaccinations, and quarantine. After recapitulating the important move of the previous chapter—the normative significance of a public health emergency—I argue that while public health ethics has often conceived of these measures in piecewise terms, a robust, securitized public health ethics will conceive of portfolios of options that include the imposition of serious liability on the state in the accomplishment of its goals. This arises from the stronger form of rights protections outlined in chapter 4, and the noncombatant analogy in chapter 5, which makes demands on states and their proxies in the achievement of their goals. I use as my example the now-ubiquitous "social distancing" measures applied during COVID-19 and show how even if we believe some kind of social distancing measures are justified, the liability required under the necessity condition of securitized public health obligates the state to provide robust supportive provisions.

In chapter 8, I consider the "front lines" of a public health crisis. Beginning with the astonishingly recent development in health security that seriously considers individuals in nonhealth service positions as "essential," and the moral implications of that in the context of the COVID-19 pandemic, I turn to an account of the responsibilities and roles of different institutional actors during a crisis. I argue that professionalized public health and medical services do in fact incur some liability in the service of defending society against public health threats. This liability is far from unlimited, but it is less sensitive to negative popular reactions against public health measures than might be initially presumed. I then turn to what I consider one of the critical elements of public health response: leadership. I argue, using the example of COVID-19, that leadership is not merely a set of personal qualities in an individual, but a normative claim about the role a person has in an institution of public health. Leadership emerges from—and in turn should inform the structure of—public health institutions, and I show how US leadership is incomplete even on the best of days, as judged not from the individuals in power but the lines (or lack of lines) of power and communication that beset the US Public Health Service. I conclude with a brief comment on the limits of that power and the role of conscientious objection and disobedience in public health.

Chapter 9 rounds out the basic argument of the book with a view to "public health peace." I argue that a central implication of securitized public health is not "war," but rather that war should be seen as the unfortunate and, by the demands of justice, rare exception to a state of peace. I then inquire as to what this peace might mean. I do so through the lens of what the public health state should look like outside of the crisis, focusing on funding and the distribution of resources and priorities. I then turn to the transition from war back to peace in public health, with a look at reparation, rebuilding, and accountability of actors during the crisis.

The final chapter is policy focused and asks the question "so what?" This chapter is a series of reflections on the state of health security as one of its practitioners, informed by the findings of this book. I present three narrative visions—stories of what a consequence of this work might be if taken seriously, for interested parties. The first vision is titled "Health Hawks, War Doves" and considers what an ambitious and comprehensive view of changing public health practice might look like. I do not attempt to estimate the actual size of the lift here, but I am clear on the contours of just how demanding this revolution might be. The second vision is titled "Business as Usual, with a Twist" and considers what the most modest view of this book's prescriptions might entail with a focus on chapters 8 and 9—which I consider the book's easiest lifts. The final vision attempts to wrestle with a persistent concern foreshadowed in this book—that the authority of the public health state might be unsalvageable. Titled "The Breakdown," I consider what a reader who is (as I am at times) deeply skeptical about the possibility that the nation-state can deliver on the demands of justice, and truly protect the public's health, might do about health security. I conclude with a comment on the relative compatibility of these visions.

2 The War Metaphor

The war metaphor is ubiquitous. It frames policy documents, international statements, scholarship, news, and opinion. In COVID-19, the "invisible enemy"[1] that was SARS-CoV-2 threatened the "[physician, nurse, and scientist] heroes on the front lines"[2] of healthcare and required "mobilizing against COVID"[3] including a "Manhattan Project for COVID"[4] to "defeat"[5] the virus over a "long war."[6]

There are other books on the role of military metaphors in a variety of settings. There are books about their relation to specific diseases, what they do to people and institutions, and the consequences of those actions. What I want to start with, however, is the idea that war metaphor is at its heart a series of choices about who counts (physicians and nurses) and who doesn't (non-"heroic" personnel such as low-paid service workers), what people really think about the reality of waging war (an epic struggle, rather than boredom punctuated by death), and what people who think about health security care about (arguably, not rocking the political boat even if it means forgoing meaningful change).

For a tight, interesting version of this phenomenon, we can look to Peter Daszak of the Eco Health Alliance. Speaking to the *New York Times* about the search for future pandemic diseases, Daszak said:

> We don't think twice about the cost of protecting against terrorism. We go out there, we listen to the whispers, we send out the drones—we have a whole array of approaches. We need to start thinking about pandemics the same way.[7]

There's a lot to unpack here. First, we certainly do think twice about the cost of protecting against terrorism: many, many people care deeply about the cost and ultimate effectiveness of US and global counterterrorism, including relative spending compared to other important social goods such as public health. And typically, the forgotten costs of counterterrorism include civilians in foreign theaters injured or killed by operations, including when we "send out the drones." It isn't clear that Daszak thinks the War on Terror is justified, but the effect is to endorse it as a template on which to build responses to global public health crises: a cruel irony given that the US, and its allies, have almost certainly lost that war.

The purpose of this chapter is to build out and describe the relationship between public and national security with an eye toward a normative argument in future chapters. That is, I show not just that there are parallels between war and disease, but that these parallels can inform how we should act in public health crises.

First, I address the obvious concern that securitizing health—turning health into a security issue—is at best a mistake, and at worst an intentional move to capture health under the rubric of national security, with all the perils that entails. Securitization theory is a broad landscape of theories, and I deal here with those elements that speak against any further comparison between health and armed conflict.

Next, I outline a series of properties that communicable diseases can possess that makes the comparison between health and security so apt. These are (1) the presence of a threat to a large number of individuals in society, and/or the continuity of society itself; (2) the requirement to mobilize against that threat being fulfilled best or only by the state; and (3) that mobilization requiring particularly weighty decisions—surrounding killing or otherwise severely limiting the life plans of individuals—to fulfill its aims. These provide a *pro tanto* reason to accept the idea of health security, though the details have to be filled out.

I conclude by examining one method by Rita Floyd, which is to consider a "just securitization" of health in certain cases.[8] I argue that this fails on a key count, which is that Floyd considers securitization a transient affair in which things come to, and cease to be, security issues. I contend that this is a mistake in the case of public health, because (1) the issue here is not strictly security, but a set of principles which public health may hold in common with security; and (2) even if public health is a national security issue explicitly, it can never be "desecuritized."

Securitization

A central criticism of health security is securitization theory and begins with the pragmatics of language. Securitization theory is concerned with speech acts that frame something as a security issue:[9] while there are a number of distinct traditions in this theory,[10] the branch that deals most with the pragmatic critique of the war metaphor is the work of Barry Buzan, Ole Wæver, and Jaap de Wilde. Securitization, they hold, casts a particular issue as a "security issue" that is distinct from normal political or policy concerns by using the language of security, threats, and vulnerabilities "staged as existential threats to a referent object by a securitizing actor who thereby generates endorsement of emergency measures beyond rules that would otherwise bind."[11] Put another way, securitization is the process by which people use the language of national security to convince each other that an issue is a threat, a critical issue for policy and politics, and one that requires expanded power and authority to address.[12]

Securitization theory typically is not an account of what security ought to be but rather a description and critique of the process by which things come to be seen as security issues.[13] The process described has its analogue in the works of J. L. Austin, whose work described three elements to speech:

- Locution: the propositional content of the act, i.e., what the words mean;
- Illocution: what kind of act it is (e.g., warning, questioning);
- Perlocution: what kind of effects the act has.[14]

Securitization is clearly concerned with the perlocution of security language: what happens when you use words to describe something in the language of security. But securitization theorists are also, I suspect, concerned with illocution. The war metaphor, among other things, is a warning to an audience. While the result is particularly important, the form of the message surely matters as well. The perlocution is that we are persuaded to treat health as a security issue; the illocution is that we are warned or urged to do so.[15]

Not all writers on securitization theory consider securitizing health to be negative overall.[16] At its most stark, however, the pragmatic critique of treating health as a security issue is more or less propagandistic. That is, securitization is the process by which security risks are *created* through the language of security. This process is rarely, maybe never, analytic: there is no principled reason why the issues we label health security ought to be thought of as security issues. Rather, the effect of the speech act itself is the process of creating agreement, justified or not, that health is a security issue.[17]

Lorna Weir has documented the rise of the language of "(global) health security" as an act of securitization beginning in the 1990s with Canadian and US efforts to define, and then incorporate into global governance, the concept of "emerging infectious diseases" and then "render WHO responsible for preventing the international transmission of emerging infectious diseases."[18] Through the early 2000s, this became a task to which WHO, driven by what Weir identifies as the interests of the Global North, responded by outlining a system of disease surveillance and control they termed the "world on alert," a metaphor explicitly tying health to security. It ultimately dovetailed with ongoing efforts to update the IHR, and after the terrorist attacks of September 2001 became explicitly wrapped up in responding to chemical, biological, radiological, and nuclear attacks. These two factors, among others, led to proposed drafts of IHR that explicitly favored a "threat-defense" conception of public health, and one that focused not on responding to endemic disease but on emerging diseases that crossed international borders. In particular, Weir rightly identifies the use of the language of threat as the language of security, rather than public health conceptions of risk.[19]

Another account of the securitization of health comes from Colin McInnes and Kelley Lee, who note that while diseases have crossed territorial borders since antiquity, their successful move into the realm of foreign policy has been achieved only recently. They identify two causes for the move in predominantly Western circles: the HIV/AIDS epidemic as indicative of novel disease threats to national interests, and fears of bioterrorism. They argue that while this has successfully connected the domains of public health and national security, this connection is in practice largely unidirectional, favoring health issues that threaten the interests of the rich, privileged economies that pioneered the securitization of health—a rhetorical move that applied national security concerns to public health institutions but not the other way around. They note, however, that foreign policy issues such as national stability and transnational criminal activity have not been singled out for their public health impacts, given the burgeoning overdose epidemic in North America at the time of their publication.[20]

Both these accounts reveal reasons to accept part of the securitization critique. First, Weir's account notes the idiosyncrasy of WHO using what we can take to be a war metaphor ("world on alert") and the language of security ("threat-defense") as a rhetorical move to generate political cachet in the international governance landscape. McInnes and Lee note that a concern about securitization is that it risks replacing the logic of public health with national security rather than linking (and, we might hope, reconciling) the two. Indeed, Weir notes that the introduction of the threat-defense conception received considerable pushback from states in the Global South, of which the most forceful is the so-called Montevideo Document produced by the governments of Argentina, Bolivia, Brazil, Chile, Colombia, Ecuador, Paraguay, Peru, Uruguay, and Venezuela.[21] That document noted that

> We propose to replace the concept of *threat* with *risk* throughout the document, especially in the definition of a *public health emergency of international concern (PHEIC)*.
> We support the definition of *public health risk* presented in the Proposal by the Chair and we justify the use of this broader concept which is more adequately suited to public health purposes.[22]

The Montevideo Document rejects the use of "threat" precisely because of its perceived ill fit with the aims of public health. Interestingly, over the next decade the attitudes of roughly half of these actors would begin to change, as Argentina Chile, Colombia, Paraguay and Peru would ultimately join the Global Health Security Agenda, arguably the first explicitly "health security" multinational agreement.

Amanda Moodie and colleagues, in their recent survey of health security, identify three major assumptions that health security practitioners make in choosing to identify health as a security issue:

1. Securitising health generates resources for responding to severe disease outbreaks.
2. Securitisation fosters multilateral cooperation on public health problems.
3. Synergy between national security and public health communities is necessary for rapid responses.[23]

They note, however, that none of these assumptions hold, and in fact often the practice of labeling a health issue one of security backfires, creating the opposite result to those assumed. Here, I describe how this arises.

First, consider briefly the United States' categorization of Ebola virus disease as a health security threat in the United States. This entailed, among other things, a large amount of basic and applied scientific research into medical countermeasures to treat Ebola virus disease; the stockpiling of resources to respond to the disease; and the generation of policy and legal tools to deal with the disease as a security threat, from surveillance efforts to restricting access to samples of *ebolavirus* under the Federal Select Agent Program.[24] Yet the background to this is that the United States saw the beginnings of the collapse of confidence in vaccinations and the resurgence of previously controlled diseases such as measles,[25] the continued tragedy of the HIV/AIDS epidemic left to fester in the 1980s, and the current over-dose epidemic catastrophe. While Ebola virus disease *is* a public health concern, it is largely not one in the US.

Second, not only does its status as a national security threat likely not serve Americans, the national priorities of the US and other developed nations in ensuring their own safety against a disease that has caused fewer than a dozen deaths in the developed world since 1974 may also have come at the cost of the public health of nations that are vulnerable to Ebola virus disease as funds were directed toward securitized diseases, while more common diseases with much higher absolute mortality and morbidity remained underfunded. Even when low- and middle-income countries have attempted to engage in their own public health measures, security may frustrate this indigenous capacity: for example, the UK has been accused of using national security legislation to prevent Western African communities from accessing their own blood for viral samples of Ebola virus disease for use in conducting research to prepare for future pandemics.[26]

This last problem dovetails with the second concern Moodie and colleagues raise: multilateral cooperation. By and large, the rise of health security has failed to make the world safer from infectious disease. This is primarily because while some progress has been made in limited areas, overall foundations of global health remain very weak. Funding for WHO, for example, remains incredibly low relative to the needs of global health. The global patent system currently stymies the creation of large amounts of vaccines and medical countermeasures under the assertion by developed nations that it is necessary to promote "innovation"—innovation that developing nations can never afford. And those resources developing nations often do have in abundance—samples of either pathogens or of plants and animals that may be reservoirs of protein and other small molecules that inspire medical innovation—are frustrated as developed countries refrain from supporting international instruments that would allow them to fund their economies and public health systems using the profits from access to natural materials.[27]

The third and final issue is most stark, and amply demonstrated through the long use of not international but domestic security as an arm of public health. The use of policing as a framework for public health has its own considerable and ugly history. Perhaps best-known outside of medical history, the rise of criminalized approaches to people living with HIV/AIDS led to a number of pernicious effects. First, laws criminalizing the transmission of HIV/AIDS or failure to disclose a person's status backfired, leading to increased suppression of HIV/AIDS awareness and education and an uptick in cases. Moreover, it had distinct gendered effects through the criminalization of women with HIV/AIDS subject to sexual violence in case their attacker contracted the disease.[28] In more recent times, the use of criminal justice institutions to address the ongoing overdose epidemic has failed to stem the rate of overdoses, and the use of prisons to house individuals experiencing substance abuse disorder has exacerbated suffering and death without any proportionate benefits.[29]

The last twenty years of international security have not helped things. Weir notes that the negotiation of securitized language in IHR occurred during the beginnings of the war in Iraq, and member states raised concerns that use of IHR to investigate alleged uses of chemical, biological, radiological, and nuclear agents could manifest in pernicious ways, including espionage.[30] This concern may have been particularly incisive given both the status of the evidence used to justify the war in Iraq and the technical dominance at the time of the US CDC, which situated it as (at least in the eyes of some state parties) the operational arm of WHO.[31] The war metaphor is off to a shaky start in part because of the history and character of wars past. To return to Daszak's comment at the beginning of this chapter: if the War on Terror is the model, it is perhaps the worst model we could choose.

The Strength of the Comparison

Securitization theory presents a significant challenge to health security. The critique is largely descriptive, asking "how have people used securitized health and to what effect?" But there are two other ways we might interrogate the war metaphor. The first is to ask, "what kinds of concepts might the war metaphor describe?" The more important sense in which we might interrogate the war metaphor is analytic or ameliorative. By this, I mean we can ask the question "To what goal should the concept in question aim?"[32]

Securitization theory will claim, and rightly, that the war metaphor is socially constructed. But if this is so, then we can inquire into what point there is in keeping such a construction around, and if there are points to which we could apply a concept like the war metaphor in order to do productive work.

The first of these alternate methods of inquiry is my method in this chapter. The study of war as a metaphor in health is hardly new. Susan Sontag's work *AIDS and Its Metaphors* is the iconic view of this area, in which Sontag describes efforts to reduce mortality from a given disease are called "a fight . . . a war."[33] There are many relationships between armed conflict and health (including medical and biological) concepts, and I won't deal with them all. I set aside, first, the work of actual intelligence and military agencies in responding to pandemic disease, such as the warnings of the danger of COVID-19 given to the US government by its intelligence community that went unheeded.[34] That is, I am not interested in health security merely as health work *done by security forces*. There may be an argument for using the armed forces in this way, but that is not my project here.

Some biological comparisons, I only deal with in passing, such as the description of patients—especially cancer patients—as "fighting" their disease, which may be interwoven with normative judgements about people's deservingness of their condition.[35] And I will largely ignore the use of military metaphors in describing biological processes, such as Ed Yong's use of T-cells and B-cells that remain after an infection as "veterans of the COVID-19 war of 2020, bunkered within your organs and patrolling your bloodstream."[36]

Rather, my focus on the war metaphor is an entry into interrogating how ideas about national security might inform public health ethics. The war metaphor describes three things:

1. the scale of the *threat* of infectious disease (or a particular outbreak) as similar to the threats that motivate armed conflict, cashed out in terms of
   - the harm they cause;
   - the psychological effects they elicit;
   - as a threat to national sovereignty, community integrity, or social function;
2. the mobilization required to respond to that threat as similar to that required by war, and its locus in *a social institution*;
3. the kinds of decisions that institution may be required to make in virtue of the exigent circumstances presented by the threat.

It is the ultimate mission of this book to determine a principled foundation for these things the war metaphor describes, and examine their prescriptions and probe their limits. Here I sketch out the features of each arm of the war metaphor to connect the ethical and political-philosophical features of public health, through this analogy, to the same features of military ethics. This will motivate further examination of the justification for the use of political power and force, broadly construed, to achieve public health aims.

Threat

In the previous chapter, I noted that President Trump invoked the war metaphor to advance a narrative of self-sacrifice during COVID-19.[37] It is not clear that this is the first American use of the war metaphor during COVID-19, but it is perhaps one of the strongest and most public instantiations of it in the early phases of the pandemic, at a time when US cases were still measured in the hundreds and there seemed a possibility of "winning" the war.

Other leaders echoed the use of wartime metaphors. In her address to the nation, Queen Elizabeth II recalled the blitz of 1940, saying, "today, once again, many will feel a painful sense of separation from their loved ones," referring to the social distancing measures enforced on the country, "but . . . know, deep down, that it is the right thing to do."[38] This depiction of COVID-19, and the measures required to address it, as analogous to the threat of Nazi invasion, frame the pandemic in terms of wartime threats to individuals and communities. The Queen even invoked Vera Lynn's anthem, *We'll Meet Again*, in her speech, further coupling World War II to COVID-19 as equivalent moments in history.

Greg Koblentz and Michael Hunzeker referred to COVID-19 as an "adversary" capable of removing a US Navy aircraft carrier from service for the first time since World War II.[39] They noted that the threat of the disease could undermine US military readiness through attrition from illness, or through the need to redeploy units to the homeland to assist in maintaining public infrastructure. But they also argued that historically, pandemics have been more deadly than war in terms of the number of lives they claim, and that if unchecked, COVID could kill more Americans than the combined death toll of post-World War conflicts.

Koblentz and Hunzeker unknowingly echoed the context framing the Tuskegee syphilis study. That work was begun due to ongoing concerns that, among other strategic issues, the emergence of syphilis outbreaks in the US armed forces could render troops unfit for duty, compromising US force strength. Resolving that concern would ultimately be the responsibility of the US Public Health Service (PHS) and US Surgeon General, who exploited African American men as a model for other populations on the racist belief that treatments for syphilis were not effective on "promiscuous" African Americans, who would thus not be harmed by their absence.[40] It's extremely doubtful Koblentz and Hunzeker intended this comparison but, as securitization theorists note, their unwitting connection to the dark history of the US PHS is not unexpected: a key effect of securitization is using the language of security to justify otherwise extraordinary or impermissible acts.

These uses reveal three separate senses in which disease poses a threat, and how that motivates comparisons to war. First, disease and war both kill, and appear to kill indiscriminately, arbitrarily, and capaciously. Michael Walzer, in introducing the "crime of war" in his foundational *Just and Unjust Wars*, notes that the basic and easy answer behind why war is wrong is simply that "people get killed, and often in large number. *War is hell*."[41] So too, then, is disease: in her *Pale Rider*, Laura Spinney describes the effects of the 1918 H1N1 influenza outbreak, mistakenly named "Spanish flu," and asks:

> How could you explain the randomness with which the disease selected its victims, if not as the work of a vengeful or vindictive force? Yes, the young and firm were in the firing line. But why was one village decimated, while a neighboring one got away relatively unscathed? Why did one branch of a family survive, while a parallel one was snuffed out? In 1918 this apparent lottery was inexplicable, and it left people profoundly disturbed.[42]

Disease, and infectious disease in particular, threatens human life and well-being on a grand scale. While estimates of the total number of dead vary greatly, World War II resulted in somewhere between 35 and 80 million deaths; the 1918 H1N1 influenza outbreak is estimated to have killed between 50 and 100 million people.[43] The worst single disease epidemic in human history then is equivalent, in lives lost, to one of the worst armed conflicts in human history. Smallpox, over the course of the twentieth century before its eradication in 1980, is estimated to have killed half a billion people—more than all wars of the same century.[44]

However, loss of life doesn't seem motivate the war metaphor by itself. Influenza claims between 12,000 and 60,000 American lives annually,[45] of an order similar to US casualties in Vietnam, at roughly 52,000.[46] However, we typically do not think of a "war on flu" in the same way we have spoken about the war on COVID-19. Even though the pandemic is much larger in terms of its death toll, seasonal influenza is a persistent enemy that we consistently fail to repel. Or so the war metaphor might suggest.

One reason we might not consider influenza an annual Vietnam is that influenza is not a discrete event, but a series of repeat outbreaks of different kinds. This claim falls short, however, given other sources of mortality such as cancer. President Nixon declared "war on cancer" in 1971 with the signing of the National Cancer Act, mobilizing the National Cancer Institute and creating the National Cancer Advisory Board, against a "disease" with a diverse series of etiologies and biological differences. The war on cancer has continued through the twenty-first century, and the incorporation of parallel metaphors such as the "cancer moonshot"—which, for those familiar with the history of the space race, know is just as militant—in more recent phases of the war. But while cancer kills hundreds of thousands of Americans per year, and even if we granted its singular nature in that "war," we don't see the war on heart disease or medical error, which cause similar rates of death per year.[47]

One possibility is that like other security threats, there is a set of events, actors, and circumstances that make us unsafe, and another set that makes us *feel* unsafe.[48] Not all of the former belong to the latter, a disjunction with important consequences. Writing in May 2020, Shad Thielman noted that by April, COVID-19 had killed the same number of people as the reported total number of Americans who died in Vietnam. Thielman's article concerns American reactions and mourning to a protracted and unjust event that resulted in the deaths of tens of thousands of Americans. Arguably, the country is as divided about the appropriate response of the US government to COVID-19 as it was to Vietnam, but Thielman points to the psychological impact of COVID as parallel to that of the war, albeit leading us there through mention of the specific number of casualties—the number of which is now in excess of any war but World War II. In contrast, fears of highly pathogenic avian influenza H5N1 led to 2005 appropriations by the US Congress that, by 2012, meant the US allocating $13 million per case of the virus in humans worldwide, an astonishing amount of money compared to the amount it spends on basic healthcare on each American.[49]

Mobilization

Another important sense in which the war metaphor applies is the mobilization of resources required to counter a threat. At times, this aspect of the metaphor is only skin deep, such as the offhanded reference in *Nature* to scientists "redeploying to fight coronavirus," referencing the reallocation of scientific labor from non-COVID research tasks to both research and development, and testing patient samples for the virus.[50] James Hamblin, writing in *The Atlantic*, described the allocation decisions made by healthcare workers around expertise and equipment as similar to those experienced in natural disaster or war, stating that while "widespread rationing by healthcare providers is unprecedented in the modern history of the United States, it is constantly happening around the world"[51]—ignoring, perversely, that rationing is widespread for many millions of Americans who lack access to adequate healthcare outside of a pandemic, and have to routinely allocate choices between care and other necessities.

On April 5, 2020, then US Surgeon General Jerome Adams entered the fray of military metaphors. During a period in which states were pleading with the federal government for access to medical equipment and testing supplies, Adams claimed that the pandemic represented a "Pearl Harbor moment," utilizing the Rosie the Riveter slogan "We Can Do It!" However, the comments were met with condemnation from state governors around the country, who noted among other things that World War II was a period of federal, rather than individual state mobilization.[52]

But the metaphor became much more literal. On April 6, US Representatives Susan Brooks (R-IN) and Ami Bera (D-CA) forwarded a proposal for a "COVID-19 Response Corps" to help stop the pandemic. The proposal was based on earlier work by the Center for Strategic and International Studies, which suggested the development of a "US Global Health Crises Response Corps" to strengthen and maintain US health security beyond what was considered a boom-and-bust cycle of preparedness measures.[53] The Response Corps, they argued, could be overseen by the Federal Emergency Management Agency in collaboration with the US CDC and PHS. While Senate Democrats enacted a bill to expand national service programs to respond to the pandemic, this bill was stuck in the Senate Finance committee. The name, however, appears to have gained some traction, used by the CDC Foundation,[54] Boston University,[55] and North Carolina state government.[56]

Mobilization in the war metaphor relies on the connection between the industrial nature of war, and modern war in particular; and the resources required to address a critical public health need, particularly a public health emergency. Public health is not cheap. Even though the adage that an ounce of prevention is worth a pound of cure definitely applies in public health, it is still costly. This cost, unlike the slick adverts of military power around the world, is largely invisible to the population.

It is not the mere cost of public health that ties together the mobilization aspect of the war metaphor. The political economy of public health means firms[57] have very little incentive to act individually to promote public health. In some cases, public health may even be a barrier to profit maximization in nonemergent contexts.[58] That is, precisely because an ounce of prevention is worth a pound of cure, the treatment of disease can be more profitable than its prevention in environments where medicine is still wholly or predominantly a profit-making entity.

Critical accounts of national security may further hold up a profit motive in war as undesirable[59] and/or unethical.[60] In a similar vein we might think that one of the strong connections between war and public health is that the incentives that drive response should be if not wholly, then substantially removed from individual profit motives. This is obviously not the case in practice—this book was written a few miles from Raytheon!—but remains a significant normative concern with which we must wrestle.

Even absent disincentives, coordination remains an issue. Public health events, like armed conflict, are often geographically broad and logistically burdensome. Substate actors may lack the power, resources, or incentives to act on a scale that actually addresses a public health need, particularly in emergent cases. One of the reasons the nation-state might have claim over public health within its borders is that there aren't other actors that have the incentive or the capacity to coordinate activities over the appropriate geographic range and population. In the US this problem is particularly acute, where fifty separate states can act autonomously without any overarching coordinating principle against a given outbreak. Public health is also a global phenomenon over which nations should have aligned interests, so this need for authority might conceivably even need to be global or at least multilateral.

Coordination problems have been a source of inspiration and criticism during the COVID-19 crisis. In March, President Trump used the Defense

Production Act (DPA) to press General Motors into the production of ventilators for use on critically ill COVID-19 patients. Designed to mobilize industrial and infrastructural resources during armed conflict, DPA has been promoted by former members of the US National Security Council and FEMA as a means to secure the necessary human and resource capital to address the ongoing pandemic.[61] However, Jared Brown notes that DPA's use during the 2009 H1N1 influenza outbreak underscored the need for reform of DPA to adequately handle pandemic disease and other threats to public health.[62] Despite this need, the ability to reform DPA has been hampered by its status as a political football, including conspiracy theories circulated during the Obama administration about the then-president's intentions to "seize control of the economy," made by a range of right-wing figures from Congresswoman Kay Granger,[63] Jim Powell of the Cato Institute,[64] to *InfoWars* host Alex Jones, among others.[65] Mobilization, like threat, is thus connected to broader normative appeals around public health and its relation to state power.

Mobilization ties to security because the kinds of threats that fall under the rubric of national security are typically those with very high costs. Because individual actors may be unable or unwilling to respond, some kind of response by the state may be warranted. This may include the state compelling private entities to reallocate resources to respond to a public health crisis, compelling public citizens to maintain social distance and break the chain of transmission, or repurposing government funds through executive power to fund a response effort. This kind of mobilization parallels what we imagine is required to repel adversaries in armed conflict.[66] There are public health mirrors to defense production, conscription, censorship, and war bonds.

High-Stakes Decisions

The third sense of military metaphor is in the decisions required of individuals and communities in responding to a threat. War is a situation in which authorities and individual soldiers must make extraordinary, even seemingly impossible decisions. Part of the impetus for just war theory is that the "crime of war" is so extreme that it may only be pursued for a just cause. Killing is almost always wrong, and so exigent circumstances are warranted to engage in individual killing in war, much less the industrial or automated carnage of modern war.

The logic of military decision-making emerged during COVID-19. Tom Frieden, the former director of the US CDC, wrote in March 2020 that America faced "a long war ahead" in fighting COVID-19. Frieden's use of the metaphor drew parallels between the strategies of waging war and responding to COVID-19. He used it, in particular, to critique the newly imposed shutdown orders around the country, claiming "strategy is important. The leading concept, now remarkably widely understood, is flattening the curve. This is an important tactic to protect patients and health care workers from a surge that can overwhelm our hospitals, increase death rates and put health care workers' lives at risk. But it is not a strategy."[67] Frieden's conclusion was that then-new social distancing measures enacted by the United States were not sufficient to ultimately deal with the pandemic in the long term but needed to adapt.

Frieden's comments emerged from a melee of war metaphors. Richard Danzig and Marc Lipsitch invoked the "long war" some two days before Frieden, laying out a plan to deal with the "surprise attack" of COVID-19: minimizing errors and uncertainties and maximizing confidence in judgments about recovery and immunity to the disease, meeting healthcare demand for COVID-19 patients over a long period of social distancing, protecting critical infrastructure that might be impacted by the pandemic, holding national elections during the pandemic, and addressing the long-term challenges for school-age children. Their central message was that the US would "[win] the war against COVID-19 as we have won other wars: by treating it as both an emergency and a long-term challenge."[68] It's not clear precisely what other wars they were referring to, if any, but the emphasis they placed on the tension between emergent response and long-term challenges will reappear in later chapters.

Micha Zenko used the war metaphor as a device of criticism against the Trump administration.[69] Zenko described COVID-19 as a "strategic surprise," which for nonnational security readers is a term of art that describes an event or development against which a nation-state is unprepared, and thus results in a sudden defeat or very high cost to repel. It is used typically to describe developments by other human actors, but dovetails with more recent concerns in the national security community about the role the changing natural environment, including emerging infectious diseases or climate change, may play in threats to US national security.[70] Zenko's articulation of COVID-19 as a strategic surprise does not necessarily mean it was *unexpected*, but rather that it is an artifact of the lack of institutional readiness we would expect in national security.

Both war and public health emergencies involve high-stakes decision-making. A classic high-stakes decision in war is how much risk to impose on noncombatants when pursuing operations.[71] If we take the killing of innocents to be impermissible on its face, and that the ends of war require us to leave open the way to return to civilian peacetime, we might think civilians cannot be attacked at any time. But the uncertainty of war, and proximity to civilian centers, means that noncombatants will ultimately be placed in harm's way. Deciding if, when, and how it is permissible to put noncombatants at risk is a difficult decision, raising questions about both the proportionality of the use of force in war, and its necessity.[72]

In the early days of the pandemic, a high-stakes decision that received considerable attention was the two-week quarantine of passengers on the *Diamond Princess*, a cruise ship docked at Yokohama.[73] Quarantine is a prototypical "liberty-limiting measure" in which the rights of individuals exposed to a virus but not yet ill are subverted by an authority in order to contain an infectious disease outbreak. In public health ethics and modern American health law, the justification for quarantine loosely parallels that of killing in war: proportionality, necessity, and the least infringing measure (in lieu of the "last resort" condition of going to war).[74]

Decision-making becomes particularly salient when considering the allocation of scarce resources.[75] While the lay public may have only discovered this problem when media began reporting on ventilator shortages in hospitals, particularly in Italy in the early phases of the pandemic,[76] the issue of allocating ventilators during public health emergencies and mass casualty events is a commonly discussed bioethical problem that received considerable attention since 2001.[77] As a general class of bioethical issues, allocation problems are some of the first encountered by bioethicists with Rescher's 1969 article "The Allocation of Exotic Medical Lifesaving Therapy,"[78] and the Seattle "God Squad" that presided over the allocation of the first hemodialysis units.[79] They are commonplace in the allocation of solid organs, and may arise for otherwise plentiful resources during emergent contexts, such as the ongoing shortage of hemodialysis units in the context of the Syrian civil war.[80]

While it has received little to no attention in the context of COVID-19 despite the use of the war metaphor, military medicine has its own logic around allocating scarce resources. Here, the logic typically is different than in civilian contexts. First, a concern in battlefield triage is if a soldier can be treated on site and returned to duty, or whether their injuries are so extensive that even with treatment they will not be able to fight. Second, doctors may experience moral tensions between allocating scarce medical resources to friendly soldiers, and to noncombatants including prisoners of war. While both groups deserve medical care, tensions may arise when there are not sufficient medical resources to adequately care for both groups.[81]

Just Securitization Theory

The above are three critical areas in which health and security overlap significantly. This gives us a reason to take the analogy between health and security seriously. But what ought we do about that?

One way, suggested recently by Rita Floyd in her *The Morality of Security: A Theory of Just Securitization*, would be to treat health security issues as times when we ought to securitize health, for a time, before returning it to its normal state. Floyd outlines a theory of just securitization, which follows along similar lines to the ethics of armed conflict doctrine of just war theory. She outlines a number of criteria for establishing the just cause for securitizing an issue, the kinds of conduct we can expect during a period of securitization, and the process of terminating a securitized state regarding an issue.[82] Might we securitize health in the same way?

I think the answer is no, for two reasons. The first and most obvious, that health security practitioners acknowledge, is that health security does not *end* as such. A public health emergency might, but this is not the same as health ceasing to be a security issue. Floyd's primary example, following her previous work, is climate change. We could imagine that at one time climate change might not be a security issue for many years, even hundreds or thousands. But health security issues arise, sometimes multiple times, within generations. They require institutional maintenance and upkeep, and in fact the lack of these, the "cycle of panic and neglect" is sometimes attributed to why they arise in the first place.

But I think the second reason why just securitization does not quite work is that we have not established that Floyd's stated goal with securitization— *making an issue the province of the national security apparatus of a state*—is what is happening here with health. There are comparisons between health and security, to be sure. But whether they actually fall under the same rubric philosophically, much less institutionally, is another matter. Nothing yet about these features of health that lend it to security make health a security issue. This remains an analogy, and like all analogies has its limits. And as I will make clear, the normative foundations on which health security relies come apart strongly from those of national security, even if they are both essential arms of the modern state.

For these reasons, we need something more. What we need is a theory of public health that operates, at times, in ways that are much like national security. But we need a theory of how and why that arises, and what form it should take.

Conclusion

In this chapter, I provided a reason to consider health to be a security issue, or like one. Following from the description of metaphors around health security in the previous chapter, I articulated the primary reason against considering health a security issue, embodied in securitization theory. I then provided three positive reasons to accept the analogy between health and security. Finally, I argued why we shouldn't see health security as mere (and transient) securitization, but something more comprehensive.

Reasons to accept an analogy, however, don't make for a set of principles to govern our conduct. In the next chapter, I examine what I consider to be the dominant framework in public health ethics, as it applies to crises that fall under the rubric of health security. I argue that these principles take us further than a mere analogy and provide us a foundation for thinking about just health security, informed by the ethics of armed conflict.

3 Reconciling Military and Public Health Ethics

In March of 2020, Texas lieutenant governor Dan Patrick made the somewhat astonishing claim that, rather than endure a complete lockdown in the face of COVID-19, many people over seventy would be willing to risk contracting the disease so as not to "sacrifice the country." Given the death rate of COVID-19 increases precipitously among those in Patrick's age group, the only reasonable message was that to protect the country, people over seventy would have to die. (Of course, at the time, as a white man in the pre-vaccine US, Patrick would statistically be half as likely to die as an African American of the same age.)[1] The trade-off presented looked simple: risk death, or stay safe at the cost of freedom, or at least freedom as Patrick saw it.

The choice between freedom and safety resulted in a hodgepodge of responses globally. The United States in particular, it appeared at times, was committed to giving its citizens the worst of all worlds. COVID-19 is, at the time of writing, certainly not gone. Social distancing measures had an initial positive effect, but for a variety of reasons most nations lacked the will and capacity to maintain this long term, leading to peaks in summer and again at the end of 2020 and 2021. In the background, the United States Congress failed to pass meaningful relief for individuals subject to public health measures, or simply caught in the disruption of the pandemic. Unemployment peaked at 14.7 percent in April 2020, though this was unevenly distributed: the leisure and hospitality industry peaking at 39 percent, part-time workers experiencing unemployment at almost twice the rate of full-time workers, teen unemployment peaking above 30 percent, and racial and gendered unemployment rates persisting over the first year of the pandemic.[2] Hospitals canceled and deferred medical procedures, and more individuals stayed away for fear of the virus. Twelve percent of Americans avoided emergency care, while 32 percent avoided routine medical care, with unpaid caregivers for adults, persons with underlying medical conditions, Blacks, Hispanics, young adults, and people disabilities disproportionately avoided seeking care for non-COVID-19 medical needs.[3] The disruption in trade and employment created a food crisis globally;[4] in the United States, 54 million people were plunged into "food insecurity" with uncertain impacts on their lives and health long term.[5] Domestic violence spiked as survivors, often women, were suddenly confined at home unable to escape violent intimate partners or family members.[6] Childhood poverty rose 10 percent over two years, according to UNICEF, an increase of 100 million children living in multidimensional poverty.[7] Vaccinations rolled out in 2021 reduced the risk of death from COVID in some countries, but the rise of escape variants of the disease brought cases, hospitalizations, and deaths roaring back—in some cases, in record numbers.[8]

Elsewhere in the world, more coordinated countries met with initial success, though some also faltered over the two-year span. In Australia, successive lockdowns enforced by police presence in some states appeared to stem the tide, and the country enjoyed a near-COVID-free life until the end of 2021 when omicron upended the nation, whose will crumbled amidst the rapid onset of the variant.[9] South Korea's rapid deployment of tests, masks, and contact tracing made it a model nation in the first year of the pandemic,[10] and while it too would experience high levels of omicron, they were lower than in other comparable economies, leading to a much slower pandemic wave and "flattened curve," to use the parlance of the early stages of the pandemic. And Vietnam's response and early success with the virus was attributed to, among other things, a long-standing engagement with public health and infectious disease that was mobilized at the right time, in the right way by government.[11]

A full analysis of every public health measure, globally, against COVID, is well beyond the scope of my inquiry. But what is important to know is that even when successful, these responses can lead to tragedy, loss, or violation. And as in war, the "toll" of COVID-19 will likely only ever be represented by the "direct" casualties, and not in the disruption and chaos that followed. Even now, it is more common to speak only of deaths or hospitalizations as the cost of COVID-19, and not, for example, the disability that arises from long-term sequelae or "long COVID."[12]

In the previous chapter I argued that far from being necessarily mere performance, a comparison between war and health captures important aspects of public health crises as people experience them. I concluded that these aspects lend themselves to a theory of just health security. Fully establishing the ethical and political-philosophical connection between armed conflict—the "war" in the war metaphor—and public health is the task of this chapter. I use the public health ethics framework pioneered by James Childress and colleagues to make this connection. This framework is not explicitly militarized, but is a foundational framework in a securitized arm of public health ethics that became important in the context of bioethics' turn to catastrophic health risks, such as the use of biological weapons[13] or the escape of recombinant organisms from high-containment laboratories.[14] It is a framework that is important to health security,[15] shares institutional origins with elements of the field, and thus is a useful starting point for investigating the possibility of just health security.

In what follows, I describe this "orthodox view,"[16] and argue that while prominent criticisms of it fail, they reveal problems that prompt a strong revision of the framework. By looking at the connection between the orthodox view and just war theory, a millennia-old framework for morally justifying acts of war, we can understand the foundations of the orthodox view in a way that gives credence to its critics and establishes the need for a fairly radical reform into a more robust theory of just health security.

The Orthodox View

Health security has an analogue in public health ethics. This view, which I'll refer to as the "orthodox" view, arises from the work of James Childress and colleagues in their "Public Health Ethics: Mapping the Terrain."[17] This is obviously not the only work that informs the current state of the art in public health ethics writ large,[18] but it is significant as one of the most cited and enduring pieces of work in the field. "Mapping the Terrain" lays out a framework for public health ethics beginning with the observation that in public ethical decision-making, disagreement on fundamental moral principles is almost certain, and it is necessary to articulate principles corresponding to general moral considerations agreed to by most.[19] The list they arrive at is one that is posited to take into account first the general preferences of individuals and respect for their autonomy, against the welfare-focused (and, they argue, paternalistic) aims of public health. The list of principles they arrive at (table 3.1) include effectiveness, proportionality, necessity, least infringement, and public justification.[20]

Table 3.1
The orthodox view of public health ethics

Principle	Description
Effectiveness	It is essential to show that infringing one or more general moral considerations will probably protect public health.
Proportionality	It is essential to show that the probable public health benefits outweigh the infringed general moral considerations—this condition is sometimes called proportionality.
Necessity	Not all effective and proportionate policies are necessary to realize the public health goal that is sought. The fact that a policy will infringe a general moral consideration provides a strong moral reason to seek an alternative strategy that is less morally troubling.
Least infringement	Even when a proposed policy satisfies the first three justificatory conditions—that is, it is effective, proportionate, and essential in realizing the goal of public health—public health agents should seek to minimize the infringement of general moral considerations.
Public justification	When public health agents believe that one of their actions, practices, or policies infringes one or more general moral considerations, they also have a responsibility, in our judgment, to explain and justify that infringement, whenever possible, to the relevant parties, including those affected by the infringement.

The status of the orthodox view *as orthodox* is first, the paper—at least as far as general frameworks for public health ethics go—is one of the most cited in the field, at around 1,000 citations at the time of writing. While it is not on a par with, say, *The Principles of Biomedical Ethics* (of which Childress is also an author), it is clearly one of the most enduring public health ethics frameworks in the field to date.

The orthodoxy of this view, however, is even more strongly established in the way the principles of the framework dovetail with other important legal and political statements about the use of force, particularly in public health. The Model State Health Emergency Preparedness Act (MSHEPA or Model Act), for example, includes principles of proportionality, necessity, and least infringement that closely align with "Mapping the Terrain." Indeed, one of the key architects of the Model Act, Lawrence Gostin, was also an author of the orthodox view, and it forms the basis for his normative justification of it.[21] It might be that the orthodox view is even an *outgrowth* of the Model Act, given it was developed in October 2001 and "Mapping the Terrain" would be published late 2002.

Likewise, the IHR restricts activities states may take to control public health risks, with the general provisions opening by noting that for public health purposes, states may require travelers, on arrival or departure, to submit to "a non-invasive medical examination which is the *least intrusive examination that would achieve the public health objective.*"[22] It modifies this, however, by noting that invasive medical examination *inter alia* shall not be required except when *"necessary* to determine whether a public health risk exists"[23] or pursuant to the general provisions. The orthodox view is also cited in WHO's documentation on global health ethics.[24]

At their broadest, the principles of the orthodox view share a language and general architecture with foundational instruments in law. Timothy Allen and Michael J. Selgelid, for example, have argued that the framing of the necessity and least infringement conditions in "Mapping the Terrain" may have been influenced by the Siracusa Principles on the Limitation and Derogation Provisions in the International Covenant on Civil and Political Rights, which includes requirements that interventions be both necessary, and use "no more restrictive means than are required."[25] Alan Sykes has suggested that the "least restrictive means" standard pervades jurisprudence, including that of the First Amendment to the US Constitution and the policing powers of the Treaty of Rome, the precursor to the European Union.[26] In their description of the creation of the MSHEPA, its authors—Gostin, above, and James Hodge, Jr.—place the least restrictive means as its lynchpin, as a means to limit the power of government to override civil liberties during emergencies.[27]

The orthodox view of public health has been subject to substantial debate, and in particular it has been critiqued in the context of health security, and its concern with both deliberately caused and naturally occurring catastrophic disease outbreaks. An initial subject of this critique is the basis on which it is consonant with other public health approaches, and in particular those that take as their starting point a firm foundation of human rights. While the human rights and health literature has as its origins the development of instruments on economic, social, and cultural rights after World War II, its "birth" has been credited to the work of Jonathan Mann and others in the context of the WHO Global Program on AIDS in the

1990s.[28] Two of the prominent goals of these movements were to (1) bring to attention the human rights considerations motivating the provision of care to people and communities living with HIV/AIDS, and (2) to push back against punitive or coercive public health measures mandating screening, disclosure, and even isolation of people living with HIV/AIDS.[29] While much of this work preceded the orthodox view, the HIV/AIDS literature, in conjunction with adjacent literature in immigrant health, global health, and harm reduction, continues to field views that form explicit and implicit critiques of the orthodox position.[30] Hodge and Gostin frame this critique in terms of the position of bioethicists and activists to portray civil liberties and human rights as inviolable over community or utilitarian concerns.[31] Importantly, Mann and his followers sometimes frame human rights as a legal instrument distinct from ethics, but here I take the two to be of a kind, insofar as human rights have, or should have, philosophical grounding.[32]

The second main thrust of the critique against the orthodox view arises in the context of the post-9/11 world in which counterterrorism has been a central pillar of national security.[33] Critics claim that the excesses of the US government in other counterterrorism responses are further repeated in developing public health policy frameworks in which individual rights are subordinated to executive power without due process. George Annas has gone so far as to refer to the Model Act, and its lack of appropriate due process and limits as it was ultimately adopted by states, as a public health version of the infamous PATRIOT Act.[34] A key move here is that even if the Model Act is in principle a well-constructed and ethically justified piece of *model* legislation, its enactment in practice is far more varied and complex. Florida's revisions to its public health ordinances in response to the Model Act, for example, included the capacity for officials to quarantine or isolate individuals for a broad array of reasons up to and including HIV/AIDS or seasonal influenza, a far cry from weaponized anthrax or COVID-19. The Floridian version of the act authorizes officials to use "any means necessary."[35] Reframing necessity from a constraint on the state, to a prerogative,[36] is a significant and frightening normative revision from the original framers of the Model Act.

Rebecca Haffajee and colleagues picked up this thread in 2014 with questions about when public health emergencies, for which the Model Act was designed, end. Noting that the majority of state implementations of the Model Act either had insufficient detail about the end of an emergency, or omitted it entirely (including my home state of Massachusetts), they write:

The notion that highly coercive measures such as mandatory blood tests, quarantines, or property seizures could be imposed for common threats without democratic procedures and full due process offends our constitutional values. The lack of clear triggering thresholds for terminating emergency powers is particularly troubling, creating the possibility that critical legal protections might be suspended indefinitely.[37]

Both the earlier and later critiques are united in the following way. The orthodox position provides a series of potential justifications for coercive public health interventions that may infringe on individual rights. However, the principles—especially when applied in practice—seem to be subject to the whims of what Annas calls "worst case thinking," in which the mere possibility of disaster is used to loosen constraints of democratic accountability in order to provide a flexible response.[38] This flexibility is vulnerable to being exploited, and critics claim is actually exploited, without sufficient justification. This tracks the main thrust of securitization theory: that it places health in the realm of national security and opens the door for certain kinds of power beyond traditional democratic oversight. The orthodox view, on this reading, does not successfully articulate a view of the scope, weight, or demand of rights to ethically justify action. In practice, it subordinates rights *ab initio* without appropriate procedural or substantive checks on power, while failing to adequately prioritize other public health needs.

The conflict between the thought of Annas and Gostin is illustrative of this debate. Annas's views are strongly representative of the critical side, while also making use of the securitization critique of the war metaphor to further his claim against the orthodox view. He claims that "human rights and health are not inherently conflicting goals that must be traded off against each other" but rather linked, citing Mann and global HIV/AIDS activism.[39] He further rejects the idea he claims underlies the Model Act that "during a public health emergency, there must be a trade-off between effective public health measures and civil rights."[40] He cites *Jacobson v. Massachusetts*, but unlike proponents of rights-infringing measures in public health he notes that the precedent the US Supreme Court used in *Jacobson* was the military draft, a wartime norm now recognized as not always required and even counterproductive.[41] Annas concludes that coercive or liberty-limiting public health measures should go the way of the draft, and be replaced with measures and tactics appropriate to the twenty-first century.

Gostin regards trade-offs between liberty and public health as fairly common, and likely inevitable. Writing on these trade-offs, Gostin variously charges of liberty and public health "more often than not they collide,"[42] and "although public health and civil liberties may be mutually enhancing in many instances, they sometimes come into conflict."[43] While Childress and Bernheim have characterized this in direct opposition to Annas,[44] this is probably overstating things. Gostin, for example, at times characterizes the trade-offs in terms of conflicts *between* rights, and in particular the clash between civil and political rights that he takes to be individualistic, and purportedly community-focused economic and social rights to health, employment, and education.[45] He also, in providing personal reflection, notes his own collaboration with Mann in informing his thoughts.[46]

However, one thing that does remain is that the principled grounding for these trade-offs is somewhat lacking. In their explanation of the Model Act, for example, Hodge and Gostin write, "In our view, individuals are not entitled to be free from every infringement of their freedoms, only those infringements that are without justification."[47] They go on to say that the state is limited in that these infringements must be the least restrictive means necessary, but do not engage in a more systematic inquiry into what the limits of those powers might look like in principle. Rather, in discussing vaccination mandates and other coercive powers of the government, they merely note that they may be required for the common welfare.[48] Elsewhere, Allen and Selgelid have noted that there also remains an ambiguity surrounding the degree to which least infringement (in the orthodox framework) and least restriction (in Hodge and Gostin, and Gostin's other writing) can be considered equivalent, all the more curious given Gostin's hand in both:

> Least infringement is thus a broad requirement that implies least restriction (other things being equal), which is a narrower corollary requirement that focuses on costs to liberty. The two are not logically equivalent: the least infringement requirement implies the least restriction requirement, but not vice versa.[49]

Gostin and colleagues' take on domestic civil rights flows into his work on international human rights. Writing in 2020, Benjamin Mason Meier and Thérèse Murphy write with Gostin that the United Nations Declaration of Human Rights recognizes that public health requires individual rights limitations provided that

> Everyone shall be subject only to such limitations as are determined by law solely for the purpose of securing due recognition and respect for the rights and freedoms of others and of meeting the just requirements of morality, public order and the general welfare in a democratic society.[50]

But we can note here that these are legal requirements, and the nature of what it means "to secure due recognition and respect for the rights and freedom for others" is still ambiguous, morally, as to the degree to which the recognition must be equal or simply proportionate remains obscure.

The contours of this debate and its responses[51] provide an opportunity and raise three possibilities. The first is the orthodox view is simply unjustified, or so mired by historical injustices that it cannot—and should not—survive. The second is the orthodox view is incomplete: while its principles reveal part of our obligations in public health, they require further elaboration in order to be justified. The third is the orthodox view is in fact correct, and its critics somehow mistaken.

The reason we cannot easily reject the orthodox view follows from the argument in the previous chapter for securitization. It is true that human rights are incredibly important, and in most cases are insensitive to welfare or other trade-offs. That, in no small part, is what it is to possess rights: to possess claims against interference, or for certain things that are insensitive to calculations about the outcomes that result from respecting those rights—at least directly.[52] But much as in armed conflict, there are rare occasions where the costs of respecting those rights are so large, perhaps even catastrophically so, that we may be obligated to infringe upon or violate those rights in aid of some much larger moral project. In this regard, pacifism is a theory of armed conflict, but one that denies this claim. But for most of us, I suspect, the question is how and when we decide to engage in those infringements, and what means we take to do so. The orthodox view recognizes this but is not alone in doing so: the same principles appear in arenas such as non-health civil rights instruments, jurisprudence, and trade law. This argument is compelling beyond its connection to national security concerns. The *relationship* may be novel, but the principles are not.[53]

We cannot, however, merely deny the critics of health security, or of the orthodox view. Instead, the orthodox position is in need of reform in important ways. And these reforms can be drawn from the ethics of armed conflict itself.

Normative Regimes, Imperfectly Realized

In the previous section I posited that the orthodox view of public health ethics was, in part, securitized. This view of public health presents as its opening gambit a set of rights, duties, and other moral considerations that inhere to individuals in a community. In particular, these considerations are claims against the state and other actors to respect, protect, or fulfill some important interest.[54] Unless some particularly stringent condition obtains, these considerations protect an individual's interests even if the consequences of doing so are sum-negative; for example, leading to less than maximized global utility. In the case of rights, they may in turn be negative claims against interference or positive claims to be guaranteed something, sometimes called autonomy and welfare rights, respectively.[55]

The orthodox view considers cases when these overriding conditions might obtain. One early example, mandatory public health surveillance, takes the trade-off between individual rights to forgo medical testing (as derivative of both general rights to bodily autonomy and privacy), and community interests in detecting and responding to communicable disease. The authors of "Mapping the Terrain" consider the conditions under which an intervention that trades off against these considerations might be justified, and the burden on the intervening actor (in this case, a public health department) to act in a certain way with respect to those whose interests are being infringed, including the risk the actor might be required to take on in executing this task.[56] Surveillance is a general ethical issue in public health,[57] but is also a feature of public health emergencies involving communicable disease.[58]

As widely accepted as this kind of conclusion might be, its normative foundations are somewhat less clear. In "Mapping the Terrain," the justificatory conditions are put down to a series of "general moral considerations" stipulated to be held by most, at least in America, and at least now.[59] Some of the authors, in separate works, provide some analysis of how we might arrive at these commitments. Nancy Kass, for example, provides a similar framework that asks

1. What are the public health goals of a proposed program?
2. How effective is the program in achieving its stated goals?
3. What are the known or potential burdens of the program?
4. Can burdens be minimized? Are there alternative approaches?
5. How can the benefits and burdens of a program be fairly balanced?

Kass, however, does not present these conditions as a set of criteria for justifying action, but rather as "an analytic tool, designed to help public health professionals consider the ethics implications of proposed interventions, policy proposals, research initiatives, and programs."[60] Her work is further derived from a version of bioethical principlism, albeit an older model reminiscent of the "Belmont Report" whose three basic ethical principles that underpin US research ethics.[61] This view holds that there are three commonly recognized general moral considerations: respect for individual autonomy, beneficence (in that report, maximizing benefits and minimizing harms), and justice.[62]

Gostin, for his part, grounds work framing his version of the orthodox view in terms of basic commitments in liberal societies. In 2003 he claimed a basic scheme of rights as constitutive of both liberal and communitarian political theories of the twentieth century. He argued that in general, public health—and in that article, responding to public health emergencies in particular—involved the trade-off between utility and/or social and economic rights on the one hand, against civil and political rights on the other. He characterized one of these social and economic rights as the right to health, against which other freedoms might be traded off to respond to, among other things, a bioterrorism attack.[63]

Gostin, however, makes a critical mistake of conflating liberal and *libertarian* thought in the same broad sphere of political theories, depicting the works of John Rawls's liberal egalitarianism and Robert Nozick's libertarian as broadly in the same family of American liberalism, and then taking the latter as his central target.[64] Along the way he accuses Annas of a kind of "left libertarianism," dovetailed into what he considers to be the core of liberalism—the limits of government interfering with self-governing behavior, claiming liberals oppose public health interventions that seek to govern fatty foods, seatbelt laws, and unsafe sex.[65] He then claims that liberals acknowledge the harm principle, associated with writers such as John Stuart Mill and Joel Feinberg, in which individual behavior that threatens others is permitted to be restricted by the state. He concludes that some economic libertarians will also permit additional restrictions based on solving economic externalities.

This basic conflation is somewhat of a problem for Gostin. While he is right that twentieth-century American liberalism is in part a response to utilitarian political philosophy, the libertarian tradition exemplified by Nozick critically arose as a response to both Rawlsian liberalism and the communitarian tradition of the same period that Gostin sets in opposition to liberalism.[66] Nozick and Rawls, I suspect, would have vastly different things to say about public health that cannot be attributed to the harm principle or concerns over externalities. Rawls, it is likely, would view public health interventions as permissible—first, so long as they respect the most expansive, coextensive scheme of basic liberties; and second, to the degree they favor the least well off as part of a scheme of basic institutions. Both are concerned with respect for persons and rights, as is Nozick, but the architecture that follows from this is quite different, in that it involves both limits on rights insofar as they are able to be jointly respected between individuals, and a distributive principle that arises from individuals' desire to maintain a fair social order.

Nozick, on the other hand, *would* almost certainly reject most forms of basic public health that relied on a redistributive welfare state. It is plausible, as Gostin illustrates, that he would condone some public health that threatens national interests to the same degree as armed conflict, or to defend against a "moral catastrophe" on par with a nuclear attack.[67] But I think Gostin overemphasizes what libertarians will condone, in part because he conflates the basic structure of libertarian and liberal thought. It is absolutely false that Nozick and other libertarians (at least Nozick himself)[68] would accept vaccine mandates, as Gostin claims.[69] And while he caveats this in terms of "high risk circumstances,"[70] Gostin is throughout referring to high risk for particular individuals, not for society-level catastrophes where Nozick might bite the bullet. Not only is anyone who has lived through COVID-19 familiar with what libertarians will or will not tolerate in practice but also, in principle, this conflation becomes a hazard for Gostin's position. This is all the more unfortunate given the divergence between Rawls and Nozick, and indeed between liberal and libertarian thought that has its direct analogue in contemporary approaches to public health ethics: Rawls's view being more or less directly translated into healthcare access through the work of Norman Daniels,[71] while a view of mass casualty response in the vein of Nozick is found in the work of Gryphon Trotter.[72]

This is important for a theory of health security because it means one of the architects of the orthodox view—and a dominant player in health security on the global stage—presumes too much first of the overlap between the political commitments of individuals, and second about the relevant options at stake when we think about responding to infectious disease using potentially coercive means. Liberal views on public health are *much* more responsive to moderate rights claims. But they are likely to be more responsive in interesting ways, privileging redistributive policies that shore up basic health outcomes, provide access to care, and increase opportunity than they are to responses to only extreme health events. They include redistributive commitments that libertarians typically lack completely. Conflating these arguably places all the political and ethical emphasis on responding to risks, and potentially shoehorning risks into threats and attributing them to individuals—just as Annas fears—rather than engaging in broader political projects to prevent these risks from arising. Liberalism is much more compatible with redistributive policies that encourage, say, sexual education and availability of affordable or even free screening than libertarianism, which is likely to favor criminalization of undeclared disease status leading to transmission of sexual diseases as a putative violation of the nonaggression principle, and avoid anything that might require progressive taxation.

The second, related concern is that even liberal thought properly defined may take divergent positions on public health, and between conventional and emergent public health decisions. Liberal thought, whether it derives from Rawlsian accounts or elsewhere, takes as its starting point that the basic freedoms of individuals are largely inviolable, even if there are some net negative consequences for doing so. A routine public health intervention that minimally satisfies the orthodox view may not be consistent at all with liberal thought. On the other hand, the use of those criteria *in extremis* may be permissible due to the emergent nature and broad threat posed by these events—though, as above, precisely what counts as emergent here will remain up for debate.

Gostin's account is explicitly concerned with emergent events, yet even here, his thinking on emergencies is still somewhat at odds with contemporary scholarship on the nature of rights. In an exchange with scholars who argue that obesity prevalence possesses the features of a public health emergency,[73] Gostin objects to the use of "public health emergency" on political and pragmatic grounds. While he denies that obesity constitutes an epidemic, much less a public health emergency, he nonetheless claims that

> whether a threat rises to the level of an "emergency" and when it ceases to be an "emergency" are both unclear. It may be more useful to think of a health threat as a continuum—as measured by the percentage of the population affected and the gravity of the harm. Thinking of an emergency as a continuum rather than a threshold makes it possible to calibrate the needed surge in resources and exercise of powers so that these are commensurate to the level of the threat.[74]

It is true that threat exists on a continuum: characterized, for example, as expected loss of life, it could be any expected number of deaths from none to all life on earth, and even all of future human life.[75] In terms of moral reasoning, if we believe some level of emergency justifies actions that infringe on rights—say, 100,000 expected deaths—though it may be wrong in some sense if we decide to act in the same way about a threat that might cause an expected 99,999 deaths, it is wrong only in a very strict and arguably morally fetishistic sense.[76] If our expected justified value for a rights infringement is 100,000 but our confidence interval ranges from 10 to 10 billion, we might be justified *ex ante* in acting even if we are later shown to have overreacted, especially if a risk is potentially catastrophic but quite rare.[77]

Yet this does not mean that from a substantive moral sense that rights violations exist on a continuum in principle, much less in practice. And this is where Gostin's account, and the orthodox view in general, arguably runs into trouble. The existence of continua does not mean that our obligations, much less actions, are also continuous in nature—the existence of shades of grey does not eliminate the difference between black and white. One central feature of nonconsequentialist moral theories, including the rights Gostin invokes in his account, is that violating them is especially bad and requires a compelling justification. Even if the threat is continuous, the consequences of acting are weighty and binary in this important sense. In almost all cases, violating rights (or duties, etc.) is worse than respecting them, and because of this we may have good reason for rights-infringing acts to be strongly protected against.[78] Being uncertain about whether or not rights infringements are justified should give us extra pause: it may generate an obligation to forgo infringement either until we have more information or even all together; and it may generate additional obligations to assume liability for our actions that constitute infringements.

From this perspective, Gostin invites precisely the challenge Annas brings. That is, the empirical claim that public health emergency thinking has largely been driven by catastrophization, fueling a cycle of "panic and neglect" to the detriment of the effectiveness, trust in, and even *presence of* basic public health, gives rise to a powerful reason to resist the idea that health security decisions that involve rights infringements can or should exist on a sliding scale. Treating all public health decisions as matters of degree, in a political sphere, leads to three possible consequences. First, it may confer excess breadth over decisions to enact liberty-limiting actions into spaces that on close analysis should not, utilizing the possibility of the worst case. Second, it may allow the decision maker dominion over a particularly vulnerable decisional sphere: in this case, public health authorities with the power to decide when to limit individual rights.[79] Third, it leads to the neglect of the positive duties of public health as an institution, and how government may be obliged to act in ways that prevent rights violations from being necessary. These correspond, broadly, to the critique of health security presented by Moodie and colleagues.

Public Health and Military Ethics

The orthodox view of public health ethics provides a guide to ethical action, but it is incomplete. It fails to consider the broader issue of how public health as a social institution ought to address limits on individual liberties, and its role in protecting rights when pursuing its charge. How then, should we proceed to think about public health? Military ethics offers a path to thinking about

1. the elements to a threat articulated by the war metaphor:
   - threat;
   - mobilization;
   - high-stakes decision-making;
2. the orthodox view in more robust terms, including
   - the justification of trade-offs between rights and threats to community;
   - the role of the state *qua* state in making decisions;
   - the way institutions ought to structure responses to continuous and uncertain levels of threat.

The combination of these situates military ethics as providing an insight into a common foundation with public health ethics.

The commonality between public health ethics and military ethics is on first blush quite straightforward. Military ethics has been principally informed by the development of just war theory over the last thousand years. A central connection to bioethics is Thomas Aquinas's reflection on the duty of Christians not to kill, and squaring that with the obligation to protect the innocent, and the resultant formulation of requiring a just cause; that the evil act not be a means to a good end, not intending the bad outcome even if one foresees it; and proportionality between good and bad outcomes.[80] This doctrine of double effect still finds use in contemporary bioethics, most famously in debates about abortion[81] and euthanasia.[82] Aquinas's insights into necessity, just cause, and proportionality were ultimately folded into Hugo Grotius's ideas of war as a relation between states and the distinction between *jus ad bellum* (the law of going to war) and *jus in bello* (the law in war), a distinction still used in ethics and international law.[83]

Conventional just war theory, unlike the orthodox view of public health, is thus divided into conditions that apply at different stages of conflict (table 3.2). *Jus ad bellum* concerns the reasons states may go to war, and

Table 3.2
The (classical) principles of just war theory

Condition	Criteria	Description
Jus ad bellum	Just cause	Armed conflict must be conducted only with just cause (e.g., as a defense against aggression, or defense of another).
	Last resort	Other forms of solution must have been exhausted prior to the declaration of war.
	Legitimate authority	The power to declare war should come from a legitimate authority empowered to make such a declaration (typically, though not always, a state).
	Right intention	Armed conflict should be pursued as a means to fulfill a just cause, and not for other ends
	Reasonable success	Armed conflict should be pursued only if the party has a reasonable chance of success.
	Proportionality	The just cause for going to war should be proportionate to the suffering war entails.
Jus in bello	Necessity	Actions in war must be necessary to achieving the proximate and ultimate aims of war (and in particular, war's end).
	Proportionality	The harm of an act of war should be proportionate to its ends.
	Discrimination	Noncombatants should, consistent with other principles, be spared the harms of war (including when doing so incurs liability on soldiers).

under what circumstances war may be engaged. Those principles envisage, broadly, a state resisting aggression by another (including defending a third party), engaging in war as a last resort once other means have been exhausted, and conducting it for the just aim of ending aggression or the defense of another. War, ethically justified, is something pursued only after peaceful relations have failed.

Jus in bello governs the use of force once war has been joined. In particular, it proscribes acts of war that are used indiscriminately on noncombatant populations, or are disproportionate, or unnecessary to ending the war. (From here on, I will frequently drop the *"jus"* as is the convention in much of military ethics.)

How does the orthodox view of public health ethics relate to just war theory? As a first step, there is a degree of homology between their principles. But interestingly, that homology arises only in terms of *in bello* considerations, leaving open a question about whether the equivalent *ad bellum* principles exist in public health (table 3.3).

Two things can be said at this stage. The first is that these comparisons need not be exact. For example, the discrimination and least infringement conditions have common features, in that they both articulate a principle of limiting the harms that certain kinds of acts cause in pursuit of the larger mission of an institution (whether winning a war or responding to a public health issue), and in particular to avoiding harming individuals

Table 3.3
Comparing just war theory and public health ethics

Temporal/contextual feature	Just war theory	Public health ethics
Before the crisis	Just cause	??
	Last resort	??
	Legitimate authority	??
	Right intention	??
	Reasonable success	??
	Proportionality	??
During the crisis	Necessity	Effectiveness/necessity
	Proportionality	Proportionality
	Discrimination	Least infringement
	??	Public justification

who are not involved or only circumstantially involved in the crisis at hand. This is why, for example, in their SARS guidance, the US CDC recommends contact tracing ahead of isolation, ahead of close contact quarantine, ahead of community quarantine, and so on.[84] It is not merely a question of proportionality—community quarantine might be proportionate in the context of a very high-risk pathogen or a biological weapon attack—but about avoiding harm to individuals who do not need to be harmed to achieve a public health goal even if this incurs greater effort or cost to the state.[85] This is similar, but not the *same* as decisions about using precision munitions or avoiding the use of air power in urban warfare to prevent civilian casualties, even if this incurs a greater burden, and lethal risk, to a state.[86]

The second thing we can note is that some principles may have no direct corollary. For example, if we consider public justification an independent criterion, it might ultimately have no analogue to armed conflict. *In bello* considerations are made in a fog of war, and moreover may require some kind of secrecy or suppression to be effective, given the importance of operational security in war. However, as I show later in this book, we might think of publicity as part of analogues to proportionality and discrimination, given the kinds of interventions public health authorities seek to achieve.

The Thin Account: Moral Exceptionalism

The comparisons between just war theory and public health ethics are significant, but that's not enough to motivate using military ethics as a basis for thinking about a reformed public health ethics. We need to explain why these principles are similar, and how that generates a reason to move from mere illustration of principles to a probative function of military ethics in establishing, critiquing, reforming, or contesting public health ethics principles. One possibility is that just war theory and the orthodox view are both examples of "moral exceptionalism," which arises when typical ethics must give way to the weight of circumstances. These frameworks could be moves to deal with cases where competing considerations override standard accounts of rights or other non-consequence-based accounts of ethics.[87]

This claim could be fleshed out first as a conceptual move similar to theories that claim rights are resistant to consequences except in very rare cases where the weight of those consequences is so great that they outweigh or override individual rights.[88] Public health ethics theories, like the orthodox view and just war theory, might both simply establish that some moral considerations (rights) are sometimes outweighed by competing considerations (some kind of threat). This is on its face broadly in agreement with the orthodox view insofar as it acknowledges a pluralistic form of ethical commitments, and seeks to balance them—but may lean more toward Annas's view if we think that the chance we are going to impermissibly violate individual rights, if allowed to do so, is very high.

As a methodological move, the moral exceptionalism claim would follow from the risk of getting our intuitions wrong about when to engage in some kind of otherwise restrictive action. This claim does not rely on the existence of rights, unlike the conceptual claim, and so is compatible with, for example, strict act consequentialist accounts of ethics. Rather, the uncertainty and potential costs of acting inappropriately through inaccuracy, inattention, or malice are high enough that a heuristic is required to determine when to act, and how. This is broadly in agreement with Kass's "analytic tool" comment, insofar as it is less about the moral commitments the frameworks espouse and more about a procedural check on decision-making.

There are reasons to reject these accounts. The first is that the emergence of just war theory was never really a threshold view, either in the early Christian or later Grotian view of the theory. There *is* a consequence-based view in Walzer's just war theory, but it is another level above the permissions and restrictions on a just war, and part of a "supreme emergency" clause in which an existential threat requires a unique and extreme response in order to preserve a community against extinction.[89] But under just war theory, the threat required to mobilize a response is not then simply a threat of harm, but a particular kind of threat that undermines community sovereignty, rights, or some other important moral consideration.[90] It is a kind of threat that constitutes a just cause for armed conflict. This is why, for example, trade wars are not reasons to go to war even if they harm nations.

Recent work in international law has established this as a component of armed conflict. Larry May has documented how even in war, the presumption that international humanitarian law is unique, or the *lex specialis*, has been steadily viewed with more and more skepticism. Writing on the problem in war, May notes "some kind of restriction on humanitarian law considerations needs to be drawn so that the entirety of the doctrine of human rights, or what is of central importance to it, is still operable for some wartime situations and other emergencies where clearly the individuals who are involved are still humans."[91] That is, even in cases of infringement of human rights, those rights *remain*, and govern our actions even if exigent circumstances justify us acting in certain otherwise impermissible ways. This is not merely a threshold view, nor a form of moral exceptionalism. Rather, we need to apply our concepts of rights in ways that remain demanding of us even in times of emergency.

The Thick Account: Common Concerns and Histories

There are better ways, I think, to account for the relationship between public health ethics and just war theory. The first is historical, and this dovetails into the second, around the kind of moral and political framework they articulate for social institutions.

The historical route brings us back through the work of the lead author on "Mapping the Terrain," James Childress. In some ways, the connection between just war theory and the orthodox view is made simple by Childress: his early work, prior to his work in bioethics, was on just war theory. Of particular interest to my project is his "Just-War Theories: The Bases, Interrelations, Priorities, and Functions of Their Criteria." Childress's work, as an opening move, picks up from something resembling the thin approach: what makes just war theory so iconic is that it looks like other cases where our duties conflict and that conflict must be resolved, including non-war cases involving the use of force and disobedience to the state.[92] This marks the approach as of a kind with public health which, while not always, does at times involve the use of force. This force exists in a broad sense: mandating certain kinds of screening and reporting for infectious disease potentially against the interests of individual privacy; or forcing individuals to stay home from their jobs, potentially impacting their and their family's future well-being. But it can also, perhaps too frequently, exist in the strict sense of physical coercion. For example, in a report to the US National Academies of Science, Engineering, and Medicine Board on Population Health and Public Health Practice, Beletsky describes how law enforcement has been mobilized in American cities to deal with the ongoing overdose crisis. While noting that police can in limited cases aid in harm prevention strategies, Beletsky argues that in practice police arrests, or syringe or condom confiscation, are counterproductive and are associated with increased levels of infectious disease.[93] This is far from the only use of state force in public health: on a basic level armed conflict and public health involve a similar in principle conflict between the use of state violence against individuals in aid of collective aims, and the need for our actions to be justified on strong moral principles such as necessity, proportionality, and least infringement conditions.

Childress's work moves beyond mere exceptionalism, however, by defining the structure of our thinking about this value conflict. Childress notes that conflicts between duties can arise even at individual levels, such as keeping promises or telling the truth.[94] But what sets war apart is the content of the *prima facie* duties that are violated, and so shape the kind of response that might be warranted. War holds the lives and deaths of whole communities in the balance, but also citizens' capacity to lead good lives, including self-determination about what that good life constitutes. Military intervention comes with a serious cost. That cost may be worth paying, but it requires special justification for the scope of duties that can be violated.

Finally, Childress sets up the central question for just war theory as—in a manner that is reminiscent of Gostin—a question of authority. That is, Childress claims the first criterion of just war is legitimate authority, claiming that "it determines *who* is primarily responsible for judging whether the other criteria are met." This is a question that is, as Childress notes, central to political philosophy, because it asks who has the monopoly on the force that war entails. This question of authority is also central to public health, given the infringements public health responses can involve and the use of state power to achieve certain health goals. Public health is thus bound up in questions of the authority and legitimacy of the state, as it is in war.

I think, however, that we should be cautious in following Childress's view of just theory into public health ethics. For one, this is an idiosyncratic view even of just war theory, which typically has as its starting point the just cause, and typically self-defense against an aggressor. Similarly, I think that public health is unlikely to be justified solely on the *ends of the institution of public health itself*, as scholars like Gostin and Hodge, Jr., do, by simply asserting the historical interest the state has in protecting public health. There is a circularity in which the institutional ends of public health are assumed, rather than justified, as a way to further justify the existence and function of that institution.

Rather, much like just war theory, health security as a particularly stark outgrowth of public health can be justified based on a threat. That is, it is the threat of communicable disease to large numbers of individuals, and even to community integrity and long-term survival, which justifies a certain kind of response. The magnitude of that threat may be great enough at times that an emergency arises in which acts that infringe upon the rights of others are justified. The structure of these rights infringements will differ from war in part because the "aggressor" is not a human agent. But even if not against an agent per se, that act of defense may infringe upon the rights of third parties in important ways. We start, as with just war theory, from the presumption that these infringements ought not happen, and then seek to examine what circumstances might trigger an emergency that leads us to act otherwise, and what our obligations are during that emergency.

This brings us to a proposed foundation for health security, and its relationship to conventional public health. Under this model, public health is first rights-respecting and rights-preserving; consistent with, to borrow a term from Rawls, a coextensive set of rights for members of a society. Conflicts do exist, but in general, according to Annas—and I suspect Gostin—promoting rights is broadly consistent with promoting public health. Where conflicts do arise, moreover, they are subject to the standard democratic process to engage in the negotiation of those rights to determine whether the scope of individual rights is indeed preserved, or if those rights need to be restructured to preserve rights for others, including the right to health.

Health security enters this equation as an instance in which rights infringement is justified in response to emergent conditions. This involves at times considerable interference with individual rights, not just of individual civil and political rights but also economic and social rights. As COVID-19 has demonstrated, infectious disease emergencies can usher in a radical change in social character, one that is scarring and even lethal. Deciding to act in this way requires special justification on behalf of the state, as does exiting it. Public health ethics currently lacks such a justificatory apparatus: it lacks its equivalent to *jus ad bellum*, though I will leave it to Latin scholars to determine what such a term would be.

This sets up the theoretic basis that informs the rest of this book: the homology between just war theory and public health ethics, commonalities in how they respond to threats, their joint grounding in the nature of moral claims against the state, and the state's role and authority in protecting its members from threats against their lives. This is partly consistent with Gostin, who derives his concept of public health ethics from broader liberal political theory. But it also attends to the concerns of Annas, and indeed of those same political theorists Gostin invokes, around the special kinds of justification that are required to engage in liberty-limiting or rights-infringing measures of citizens. This results in a framework that takes both views as partly correct, but in specific and complementary ways. What is missing is the normative framework to understand why conflicts arise, and how to justify using force, direct or indirect, to maintain public health.

Objections

Three objections are foreseeable in making the connection between military ethics and public health ethics. The first, familiar to much of bioethics, is: So what? The connection is interesting, but it doesn't necessarily give us much more out of public health ethics. But military ethics has two advantages on public health ethics that make it a useful resource. First, but weakest, is that compared to the half century or so of modern bioethics—only loosely connected to ancient medical thinkers—military ethics is an extremely long-lived discipline. Tenacity hardly tracks validity, however; compared to the age and volume of public health ethics and health security scholarship, military ethics has an extensive and deep philosophical foundation from which to work. It has moreover considered issues of rights infringement in incredibly granular detail, including the kinds of liability rights *infringers* retain when they act in certain ways.

A second response is that recent work in just war theory has connected justice issues between the conditions that lead to war, its declaration and conduct, ending, and ultimate resolution. This provides a connective framework over which we can lay the relatively narrow ethics of liberty-limiting measures in public health ethics and conceive of it as continuous with issues including social determinants of health, routine disease surveillance, public health emergencies, and what rebuilding means after a pandemic. This allows us to view questions of liberty-limiting measures in public health not as mere questions of proximate justification, but ones of political philosophy and distributive justice as well.

The next objection concerns the kind and scope of the violations a state inflicts during different crises. Surely, one might argue, the kind and scope of the violation in public health is rarely if ever as serious as seen in war, in which thousands if not millions of people die due to *intentional* killing. There is simply no comparison to public health, which at worst deprives individuals of civil and political liberties but not their lives.

The easy response to this is simply to deny, as I have, that public health never entails the intentional, or at least reasonably expected loss of life. But

I think we could do better. A central character of civil and political rights or liberties is that they are resistant to consequences because they are essential to the self-governance of individuals in communities of equal respect.[95] So the fact that someone has not died is in some ways dismissive of the kind of infraction that occurs when civil and political liberties are undermined. These conditions are frequently thought of as preconditions for a good life, and while contested it is not the case that they are less serious, in principle, than one's life. The ethics of war considers likewise not just wars of annihilation, but conquest and colonization; punishment and terror. Wars where few or no soldiers die can be incredibly harmful to communities; conversely, poorly or unjustly pursued public health policies don't have to use guns to kill people or maim whole communities.

In another sense, the infractions may be all the more serious if the public are by and large innocent bystanders in many, if not most public health emergencies. Even if they resist public health orders that tend to be effective, the citizens of a state are individuals to which a state has a fiduciary duty more than it does enemy combatants or citizens of other nations. As I will establish in the next chapter, the enemy is the disease condition identified as serious enough to warrant a public health action. Public health actions are analogous to military actions that cause high levels of "collateral damage" against the state's own citizens. In war, even the permissibility of killing other combatants is neither straightforward nor obvious; how much more for acts that might harm one's own citizens? Thus even nonlethal rights violations could be very serious as a result.

The final objection is that the nature of public health is constant, where wars are discrete. Communities are always at risk of disease and other public health threats, where war is (the war on terror notwithstanding) a discrete circumstance. The response to this is the two elements of the common foundation I have established. Wars are sometimes discrete, but they can also be continuous with the politics of states. Public health emergencies, I will argue, can be viewed as a continuation of the largely peaceful but turbulent politics of health. Engaging in the process of securing our health against threats, and treating each other's health with respect, is indeed constant. But so is preventing war. Diplomacy and other means of preventing war are as important to an account of the ethics of armed conflict as the proximate ethical decisions behind killing. The state imposition of liberty-limiting measures, or measures that violate our duties to each other, requires a special kind of threat. Public health is indeed constant, but some instances of public health break away from the usual order of things to become emergencies.

This returns us to the tension between Annas and Gostin. They illustrate, to me, points on a continuum similar to that we find in military ethics between pacifists who think war is never justified, and political realists who think war is totally continuous with politics as usual. So too in public health we may have, in principle, strong views on health and human rights that always forbid infringements on rights, compared to other views in which rights violations are simply the practice of justified public health in the name of the common good. I have argued that Gostin is not a realist in this sense about public health, but the conflict between these two demonstrates the deeply contested question about how often public health conflicts really arise, what causes them, and what we do about them. The account I have given follows the view that just war theory is a response to pacifism, seeking to start with the presumption that infringing on rights is impermissible, and showing in what cases that presumption can be overridden.[96]

Conclusion

In this chapter, I introduced the orthodox position as a securitized view of public health and defended an ethical framework for public health as an institution that may at times infringe on individual liberties. I identified the central debate, using Annas and Gostin as examples, about how often these liberty trade-offs need arise, and related this to the just war tradition. I then articulated the connection between military and public health ethics, and why a thick account of this connection provides a way forward to resolve the debate and come up with a more robust ethics of public health.

Having done that, the first order of business is to fill in some of the gaps in table 3.3 about when a state may engage in liberty-limiting measures on its own population in the name of public health. This requires first establishing the nature and range of public health threats, their impact on communities, and how these threats might engender a response. It then requires a criterion for when a public health emergency may be declared, and a view of legitimate authority. This will establish the equivalent of *ad bellum* considerations of public health before we move into deeper analysis of other elements of public health ethics using military ethics as a guide and source.

4   The Impersonal Account of Disease

Of all the events of the COVID-19 pandemic to date, perhaps none were so chaotic as when on October 2, 2020, the *New York Times* among others reported that the American president, Donald J. Trump, had been diagnosed with COVID-19. Within that news lay the implicit tension for some: "The president's result came after he spent months playing down the severity of the outbreak that has killed more than 207,000 in the United States and hours after insisting that 'the end of the pandemic is in sight.'"[1] What came next seemed bizarre, even deranged to some. The president issued a series of televised statements claiming his imminent recovery; posed as if working at the Walter Reed National Military Medical Center, typically responsible for treating the president as the commander in chief of the US armed forces; and then a car ride through Washington, while still ill, in the presidential motorcade—vehicles sealed against chemical weapon attack, and thus unable to vent air or in any way reduce the risk the president's illness posed to Secret Service personnel. The president, moreover, had been on the campaign trail, and reports trickled in over the weekend of tests not taken, quarantines and isolation broken, and social distancing measures unobserved.[2]

Commentators and the public who, rightly disdainful of the president's actions, advocated criminalizing or otherwise holding accountable individuals who intentionally imposed others to the risk of infectious disease. Physician and onetime congressional candidate Dena Grayson claimed that Trump "knowingly expos[ing] hundreds of people to the deadly coronavirus on Thursday" had committed a crime and that the president should be charged with reckless endangerment.[3] Anne Margaret Daniel, a professor at the New School, implored the governors or Minnesota and Ohio to bring legal action against Trump for the felony crimes in those states of transmitting an infectious disease.[4] Actor John Cusack promoted the view that "in a democracy, Trump would be charged with a violent felony."[5]

The calls emerged within the larger context of proposed criminalization, and ultimately militarization of COVID-19, spurred by anecdotes of individuals threatening to spread the virus to others,[6] and reports that terrorist organizations had considered spreading the virus.[7] Earlier in the year, Deputy Attorney General Jeffery Rosen had claimed that the virus that caused the disease appeared to meet the statutory definition of a biological agent, as used in US law codifying the Biological Weapons Convention.[8] This took COVID-19 beyond the criminalization of HIV/AIDS common to thirty-seven states in the USA,[9] and into considerations of national security. It arguably signaled the return of the weapons of mass destruction (WMD) aspects of the War on Terror to US soil in the form of considering an infectious disease state equivalent to a malevolent actor in possession of a biological weapon. Critics—including the author—replied that the criminalization of disease had, almost exclusively, resulted in more harms than benefits. Those harms, moreover, were not borne by presidents or rich, white businessmen of his ilk. Rather, they were borne by the vulnerable and marginalized—as author Laura Flanders wrote, "If the Donald was a poor man, poorly defended and in poor health, there's a good chance he'd be facing criminal charges."[10]

The identity of a belligerent has critical normative significance in a just theory of health security. First, even in war with humans, what we can do to enemy combatants is typically regarded to be less constrained than what we can do to bystanders in pursuit of our enemy.[11] So knowing who the enemy is, and defining them in a justifiable way, determines the moral permissibility of the kinds of acts we can make that violate individual rights.

Second, and critically, the identity of the "enemy" gives us insight into the appropriate structure of health security. A common historical theme in health security is to prepare for both naturally occurring and deliberately caused disease outbreaks in the same way: allocating funds to predict, surveil, and respond to disease outbreaks; structuring research around small groups of high-impact low-probability pathogens; and investing in public-private partnerships to incentivize the development of medical countermeasures. But rarely do we see expanded universal healthcare, investment in health systems that combat high-incidence as well as high-impact diseases, strengthening of our existing international health governance, or addressing the ongoing risks of climate change. This gap has been viewed with intensely critical eyes from securitization theorists and adjacent scholars,[12] but the precise reasons *why* we should avoid this turn, and what role the norms of national security have in public health, are not well explored.[13]

In chapter 2, I provided three primary motivations for treating public health as a security threat, motivated by the "war metaphor," which provided an analogy between public health and armed conflict. Those motivations were:

1. The threat of infectious disease in terms of
   - the harm it causes;
   - the psychological effects it elicits;
   - as it alters community integrity, social function, and even national sovereignty;

2. The mobilization of resources (including people) and logistics required to respond to that threat, including the requirement for a separate *institution of the state*;

3. The nature of the decisions required by that institution, or its agents, to prosecute their justified aims.

In this chapter I address the first motivation, and flesh it out. The central purpose of this chapter, in building a theory of just health security, is to mount an argument for what I call an *impersonal account of disease* as the appropriate target of public health responses. On this account, the "enemy" in public health, properly defined and justified as a state institution, is the causative agent of disease. In defense against pandemic communicable diseases—and in keeping with this book's central topic—this causative agent will be a virus, bacterium, fungus, prion, or some other microbial organism. But other critical public health concerns arise from other nonhuman, impersonal sources, such as environmental pollutants or natural disasters. Importantly, humans on this account are often bystanders to this threat, and even when they not are not relevantly liable to harm by the state.

My aim with this account is to derive an account of *threat* that overcomes the more extreme realist leanings of health security. The normative and conceptual apparatus of national security is dangerous, as securitization scholars show, precisely because it creates an "us versus them" mentality that harms and marginalized communities[14] and weakens public health cooperation as nations seek to protect "us" against "others."[15] It generates, through intent or neglect, policies that frequently increase public health risks rather than lessen them. But more, it generates an assumption that far from the much more demanding calculus of infringing on the rights of individuals only in dire circumstances, those rights are easily overridable because citizens are the threat to public health.

In what follows I argue that, like war, what motivates securitized public health responses is the scale of death and disruption disease involves. I then address one important account of threat in infectious disease, the "patient as victim and vector" view forwarded by Battin and colleagues.[16] I argue that this view first mistakes, or overemphasizes, causal contributions to harm as tracking *responsibility* for that harm. Second, it mistakes responsibility for imposing risk as *liability* for a coercive or dominating defensive response by another. Finally, the patient as victim and vector makes too much of the "relationality" between individuals, and—in a related but distinct way to the view of public health ethics that motivated Childress and colleagues, as I addressed in chapter 3—would better capture the morally relevant features of responding to infectious disease outbreaks understood in terms of domination, which changes the calculus of our response.

In almost all cases individuals and communities that are causally implicated in the spread of communicable disease are not necessarily *liable* for their actions. Drawing on the literature in the ethics of armed conflict, I contend that what generates the right to a defensive action is a responsible threat to an agent. I then argue that in the context of infectious diseases, specifying individuals as responsible threats is either (1) epistemically implausible, (2) misses a sizable chunk of what we care about in health security; (3) is ethically unjustified, or (4) misses the point from the perspective of public health response. While there are cases in which individual threats might motivate public health response, they are quite a bit rarer than is supposed, and not straightforwardly individuals with disease themselves. Rather, the threat of infectious disease is by and large best characterized as the threat of the causative agent of disease. I argue that because of this, we should take rights infringements of individuals incredibly seriously, given that individuals themselves are not threats, and thus should not incur the kinds of harm a public health emergency response can entail. This does not rule out public health acts, it but raises the bar to action because it must be a "least-worst" response, rather than one where individuals have become liable to response because of a positive reason to act against them.

I conclude with applied cases of this account of health security. First, I examine the role disease surveillance can play in preventing the emergence of disease epidemics and discuss how a non-liberty limiting account of surveillance might be constructed, including the use of ecological surveillance. I then turn to questions of failures to act in responding to a public health need as a source of health injustice, and the relationship between the *ad bellum* last resort condition and modern public health ethics. I conclude with a view of what I consider the primary objection people will have to take into account, those cases in which human actors do function as agents of disease, as a way to tightly define the scope of our concerns about public health threats *qua* human threats.

The Threat of Disease

In chapter 2, I claimed that the threat infectious diseases pose might warrant a securitized approach to public health. That threat may arise by virtue of the harms posed to or expected to threaten the public's health. It may also possess some psychological features that indicate it is a threat, such as a sense of immediacy or exigency posed against a community. Finally, the threat may arise in terms of a threat to community integrity or even national sovereignty.

When thinking about the moral justification for health security, with a focus on infectious disease in particular, threat is a good place to start.[17] Infectious diseases can cause public health crises on an enormous scale. This is why, for better or worse, we declared war on AIDS, which has killed approximately 40 million people worldwide since the beginning of the epidemic.[18] It is also why we declared a smaller defensive response against Ebola virus disease, which killed 11,000 people in West Africa and upended the economic and social conditions of three vulnerable countries.

But I have yet to see someone declare war, say, on road injuries, which kill more than a million people a year worldwide.[19] Road safety is surely an important and worthy topic of public health, and it does cause large numbers of deaths. But it seems strange to declare war against road fatalities. This certainly doesn't mean it is impossible, but I take it as indicative that the wars we declare on health issues are often (though not always) infectious diseases because of the scale, exigency, *and* overwhelming nature of those outbreaks.

Mere death or disability does not always engage the kinds of normative claims with which health security is concerned—even in infectious disease. We have not, to echo a claim made by conservative commentators in criticism of COVID-19 public health metaphors, declared war on influenza. This is despite influenza being a disease that in 2018 caused 35,000 deaths in the United States: when the American Medical Association "accepted the challenge to be in the forefront of [the] war on AIDS" in 1988, 16,602 deaths were attributed to HIV/AIDS.[20] It is not my purpose at this time to question whether or not we ought to have mobilized the war metaphor against HIV/AIDS, but it raises the question of "why the difference?" And *should we*, if we are justified in declaring war or mounting a securitized response to AIDS, make the same declaration on influenza?

The answer, I suspect, is partly in the second way that threat manifests—though for the wrong reasons. HIV/AIDS tapped into a deep concern and psychological vulnerability, but too little and too late. While the US government ignored HIV/AIDS, infamously to the point that President Reagan failed to mention the disease until the end of his administration, its increased attention tapped into two forms of psychological insecurity. The first was the totally justified fear by the LGBT community ravaged by the disease, whose activism turned that fear into direct action to compel the government to notice and address the crisis. The second was highly selective fear of HIV/AIDS among the "innocent," and in particular, individuals receiving blood transfusions. The wider public fear of AIDS that motivated the War on AIDS was, on most accounts, a reaction to a single "H," hemophiliacs (and other receiving regular transfusions), where homosexuals, heroin users, and Haitians would not motivate America to act on a disease epidemic.[21]

The psychological aspects of insecurity are neither a necessary nor sufficient condition for identifying a health security threat. Threats need not be recognized as such to kill you. I may be oblivious to all kinds of danger—such as the day-to-day risks I take on the road—that nonetheless are grave threats. A belligerent human aiming to harm you may ambush you because of the advantage conferred by the element of surprise. Conversely, I may have all kinds of deep fears about things that are low-level threats (e.g., the threat of international terrorism relative to domestic hate crimes), or are even totally fictional (e.g., the "Satanic Panic" of the 1980s).[22]

The third and final criterion is community integrity. Not all disease risks, even those that are very serious, threaten community integrity, even where the morbidity and mortality of a disease are very high and very costly. The cost of Alzheimer's disease is very high, estimated to cost up to $2 trillion annually worldwide by 2030.[23] However, due to its concentration at the end of life it is unlikely that the high cost of that disease ultimately threatens the internal or external function of a community, much less state. High costs, in particular, are able to be borne under a public health state through progressive taxation mechanisms, and the appropriate financing of health.[24]

Other health crises, and in particular rapidly evolving infectious diseases, might threaten communities just because their death toll is concentrated in particularly devastating ways. Famously, the 1918 influenza epidemic, compared to seasonal influenza, disproportionately killed the young.[25] The AIDS epidemic was highly concentrated in marginalized communities, including the LGBT+ and sex worker communities. And a *Pro Publica* investigation in 2020 highlighted how the COVID-19 epidemic's disproportionate toll on young Black men has hollowed out communities around the United States. In this latter example, investigation showed that COVID-19 was often the final blow in a combination of institutionally racist policies and treatments, additional and systemic public health risks, and lack of access to care imposed on young Black men, weathered by resilient people but making them vulnerable to the SARS-CoV-2 virus and the disease it causes.[26] In a similar way to the effects of smallpox on Indigenous communities during the colonization of North America, what constitutes a catastrophe from which communities may never fully recover can be local, and proximate, rather than a more obvious ultimate and globe-spanning kind of catastrophe.

Because of the conflicting meanings of "threat," then, it is important to clarify what the appropriate locus of threat is. To start, while there is a relationship between community-level risks and individual risks, a "public health threat" does not obviously track mere individual risk. Public health is, at its best, a collective endeavor pursued to promote the health of communities. So even if the most direct causal effects—morbidity and mortality—inhere to individuals, its effects and our responses are often at the level of level communities. COVID-19 is a great example of this kind of threat. Individuals die of COVID-19 like any other respiratory illness, but the pandemic has also disrupted communities, made international travel unsafe, affected trade, put people out of work, and stressed social safety nets beyond breaking point. This stress, moreover, has affected not just those affected by COVID directly but those who have missed out on access to housing, social services, employment, and medical care as secondary consequences of social disruption. This kind of threat is large in magnitude, and is, moreover, coordinated in the sense that COVID-19 is a pandemic with a coherent etiology.

What makes a threat special ethically, however, is that threats motivate a defensive response. This may be defense of oneself, or another. The language of threat, moreover, is not unknown to public health. In the United States, it is described in *Jacobson v. Massachusetts*:

> Upon these principles of self-defense, or paramount necessity, a community has the right to protect itself against an epidemic of disease which threatens the safety of its members.[27]

That is, a threat to community engenders community self-defense. But even if this is a universal idea, and not simply an artifact of American legal reasoning, it broaches the question of against whom, or what, we are defending. In the ethics of armed conflict there is broad agreement that an unjust threat against our lives—including a conditional threat, like an army threatening us[28]—permits us to engage in a proportionate and even lethal response. In the same way, just health security needs a referent: the thing that is *threatening* us.

In classical, conventional war, the threat is that of aggression, often between states.[29] That aggression prompts a reaction of self-defense, or defense of another through armed conflict, in which the military representatives of a belligerent state are subject to lethal use of force until peace is achieved.[30] But the literature on self-defense and threats is considerably more complex than that, and its principles may be applied to non-responsible threats—threats posed by actors who do not intend and may not even have a choice but to impose them[31]—and even nonhuman threats such as the threat of planetary destruction.[32] So there remains an open question about what it is that causes the threat that motivates our ability to defend ourselves against the threat of infectious disease.

Misclassifying this threat, moreover, can have serious consequences in practice. Annas identifies this in his analysis of "worst case thinking,"[33] focusing only on a prescribed set of actors and disease states and design policies in turn, which overemphasize these at the cost of other public health needs. Alternately, mischaracterizing the threat as human may lead to the worst impulses of human action, as individuals are vilified for a disease over which they have no control—revenge described as policy. In either case, these mischaracterizations either marginalize or neglect vulnerable people. In the case of COVID-19, these practices have arguably failed in their task of protecting the world against a naturally occurring pathogen, while many billions of dollars of money in the developed world have been spent on homeland defense against much rarer pathogens such as anthrax attacks and Ebola virus disease, which have killed in the tens of thousands in the last decade, almost all of them in the context of a single outbreak in Western Africa.[34]

This might leave some to resist the idea of threat altogether as useful in public health. Such a move might be part of a larger abandonment of health security, or simply a partial rejection of its completeness. This is not without cause: securitization theorists will highlight damage that arises from treating people who suffer from disease as threats. The AIDS crisis I have already described is replete with unethical and unjust behavior that arose first from willful neglect of the crisis due to its association with gay men, and later the criminalization of AIDS status as a regressive policy that harmed meaningful, rights-respecting public health interventions.

I think, however, that an analysis of threat can serve two important roles. One is to play a negative role, in which we dispel dominant conventions around the locus of threat in health security as individual humans. The other is to play a positive role in identifying what it means for a nonhuman entity to be the appropriate locus of threat in health security, and what this means for public health emergencies. I deal with each in turn.

Victims and Vectors

For my negative project, I'll use an influential view on individual risk and threat of infectious disease called the "patient as victim and vector" view developed by Margaret Battin, Leslie Francis, Jay Jacobson, and Charles Smith. As one of the first comprehensive works on ethics and infectious disease, it is important both for its historical position written after SARS, H5N1, and the identification of extremely drug resistant tuberculosis, but prior to the H1N1 2009 pandemic. It is an early text identifying bioethics' lack of attention to infectious disease as an important topic.[35]

The patient as victim and vector view gives a simple, clear picture of threat in infectious disease: individuals are both victims of a disease and vectors of its spread. The authors state that individuals thus are at least partly blameworthy for disease transmission, and thus also partly responsible for preventing transmission events from occurring. In discussing responsibility for infectious disease transmission, they write

Deliberately sneezing on one's competitor, having sex when one is aware of the possibility of transmitting disease, like chlamydia or syphilis—these are (ir)responsible acts. Similar notions of responsibility, praise, and blame apply to them, as the reckless acts that persons at risk: leaving toxic waste near a playground, having sex without protection against unwanted pregnancy, and so on.[36]

That is, we are responsible for our acts on everything from a deliberate sneeze to sex, if there is a possibility of transmitting disease. They conclude that even in unaware acts of disease transmission, we may still make choices in our lives that expose individuals to risk even if we are not aware of our infectiousness or disease state.[37]

The authors go on, however, to note that because of the complex webs of disease transmission, there is no "source" and no endpoint for disease transmission. Humans are described as "way-stations" and "launch-pads for infectious diseases. When considering knowing whether we can foresee our disease state or our chance of transmission, further, the authors claim

> The metaphysical status of human beings as individuals—their physical as well as social *locatedness*, their *embeddedness* among others who are also sway-stations and launching-pads for dangerous as well as benign microorganisms—cuts against binary judgements that people either are responsible or not responsible, blameworthy or not blameworthy.

They claim, then, that individuals are embedded in a complex web in which their responsibility for disease transmission is offset by their ability to blame others for giving them a disease in the first place. Because of this, individuals can justifiably be imposed upon to prevent these interactions, including in ways that cut against their self-interest or their civil, economic, and social rights. But this must be done, the authors claim, always with the additional "perspective of the patient as victim." Following on from Rawls's famous thought experiment in which hypothetical members of a society are asked to identify what arrangements of institutions they prefer, Battin and colleagues argue individuals deeply uncertain about their status as either victim or vector will adopt a "we are all in this together" perspective, striving to do the best, as a matter of solidarity; that is, maximize the minimum for each and every one—rather than generating a better average—with respect both to our susceptibility to disease and what is needed to reduce the overall burden of disease.[38]

I will leave the authors' account of Rawls, and how their conception of threat fits into a larger political philosophy of public health, for the next chapter. For now, their conception of public health threat is my concern as it captures some of the intuitions people seem to have around threat and infectious disease. It provides a view of the relationship between risk and threat in public health: that individuals are constantly aggressor and defender against an onslaught of potential infectious risks.[39] It also articulates what I think many would find a plausible view of that threat and our response to it: that when individuals threaten us, they waive certain rights not to be treated a certain way. The constancy of these interactions does a lot of work here, by creating a presumptive case for regarding ourselves as potential disease transmitters and receivers, and thus giving us no reason not to act as if we were a risk (and at risk).

This view, however, does too much on the one hand and not enough on the other. For a start, it is simply empirically false that, as the authors describe it, there is no beginning and end to infectious disease. This is true perhaps for some diseases, but certainly not others—and certainly not the ones that health security typically regards as threats. Even the examples that are used by Battin and colleagues—HIV/AIDS, tuberculosis, influenza—are all zoonotic pathogens. They arise in animal hosts and transmit to humans. So, unless Battin and colleagues have an account of responsibility in minds for poultry, cattle, and great apes, their account is empirically unsound for a great many infectious diseases. Diseases do come from somewhere.

I imagine that Battin and colleagues would reply that while this is true for any one infectious disease, the "web of disease"[40] writ large is the basis for their theorizing. But if we take this tack, we get something that looks more like a social scheme of risk sharing, than one in which arguments from responsibility or threat are strictly necessary. Individuals might engage in socially sanctioned activities that involve mutual risk impositions *without giving up their rights* in any meaningful way. We all drive on the roads and risk each other's lives every time we do so. While we are responsible for harm and may be responsible in a causally and even ethically meaningful way, it does not involve a strong waiver of our rights. In fact, access to the road as part of a scheme of social sharing of risk might constitute a *promotion* of our rights to movement and mobility. Instead of leaving people to fend for themselves and/or simply punishing noncompliance, we have constructed broad (though arguably neither broad nor strong enough) regulatory systems to cover insurance, licensing, road safety, traffic data, highway maintenance, and so on. Car crashes impose a serious risk of death, and at more than a million deaths per year worldwide, they are as great a source of mortality as many infectious diseases. Yet we do not presumptively lock up individuals on the suspicion they may cause a car accident to another or teach another to drive as recklessly as they can. Nor do we hold them to be threats at every turn.

The distinction between road safety and infectious disease, moreover, is not totally explained by the capacity of onward transmission of infectious disease—tuberculosis can spread rapidly in resource-poor settings, but its ability to reproduce in developed nations, the primary target of Battin and colleagues' analysis, is quite limited. When describing the forced isolation of a homeless man, Mr. K., the authors go so far as to say that the difficulty is not "whether," but "how" compelled isolation should occur.[41] But why should this be the case? We might impose a financial burden on Mr. K. or others buying a car, or an educational burden in getting a license, but we again do not presumptively restrict a major liberty like freedom of movement on the basis that they may at some future time kill someone. And—in general terms, as a statistical member of the United States, in which his case is set—he is much more likely to kill someone with a car than he is with an infectious disease, at least outside of a major crisis like COVID-19. Note, further, that I'm not saying we shouldn't isolate some kinds of patients, even forcing them to be so. However, the web of prevention model doesn't account for this in the right way.

The web of disease account by Battin and colleagues entails a threat-based analysis. In writing about pandemic responses such as community level quarantine, Battin and colleagues argue that personal security for quarantined individuals is important:

> A common social response by people who feel threatened toward people they view as threats is to try to destroy the threat by driving them away, harming, or killing. These may be understandable and even justifiable responses to aggressors of various sorts. But to regard people who have communicable infectious diseases in this way is to regard them as vectors only, and to overlook that they are already victims as well. Infectious vectors are not only aggressors—if they even can be called that—but also people themselves under threat.[42]

This explicitly identifies individuals with communicable diseases as threats. And importantly, it does not *deny* they are threats, but rather says that our responses to threats, while justifiable in other cases, are not justifiable in communicable diseases because individuals are also victims.

But what comes of this double "threat-and-victim" analysis is mysterious. Just because someone is themselves under threat does not necessarily undermine our justification for exercising permissible self-defense, even lethal self-defense. This is the heart of the justification for killing in war. Just because I am under threat by person A does not mean that the threat I pose to person B is lessened or mitigated. There might be other reasons to refrain from harming me—such as if I am a soldier engaged in a just war[43]—but the mere fact that I am similarly under threat does not obviate the threat I pose to others.

We could construct an account of individuals with communicable diseases as a threat, but it is far more restrictive than Battin and colleagues admit. More often than not, individuals infected with a communicable disease pose what we might call a "nonresponsible threat." That is, they unknowingly threaten to harm others in a way for which they are not liable and are in no way morally responsible.[44] The classic example given here is that of a man pushed from a cliff by a third party and falling toward me. Due to a lack of time to react, I will either be killed (and the man will live), or I can open a large umbrella and impale the man on it. Jeff McMahan points out that while there is a strong intuition that we are justified in enacting defensive harm against nonresponsible threats, we lack good reasons to do so. Importantly, threat has not violated our right not to be harmed—insofar as a right is something we have against others that means they are constrained in their behavior, we cannot be constrained in our behavior when that behavior is something we have no control over. I have a right violated by the villain who pushed the man off the cliff, but not the man himself. He is equivalent to a bystander in terms of my right to a defense response based on *his* liability as a threat.[45]

An extension of this example would be a kind of iterative "falling man" case. Instead of one falling man, we could imagine a falling man has been knocked off the cliff by another falling person on a terrace above, and they by another, and so on. Much like the spread of infectious disease, there is a sequence of causal events that make the falling individuals all threats to the person immediately next in the sequence. But at no point have any of them become liable for their actions, and thus they have not given up their rights against harm. My justification, and indeed anyone's justification to exercise self-defense against these threats, is not "balanced" by the victim view, in this case either.

In a similar way to the falling man, in most cases of communicable disease an individual with a disease is not morally different from a bystander who poses no threat at all. In both cases, the threat exists, but the individual hasn't forfeited their rights. Individuals with communicable disease are then more analogous to noncombatants in a war zone. They may at times pose nonresponsible threats to others, but this alone does not give us a justification to harm them in return, including by violating their rights. Rather, we require an argument in which the harms that we are preventing in responding to a threat are proportionate to the kinds of harm we are inflicting on innocent threats. But note that this kind of "least-worst harm" argument does not depend on liability, but on proportionality, necessity, and last resort alone.[46]

An easy objection to this is that many individuals perform acts that arguably and knowingly put others at risk. For example, they go to work while sick knowing they could spread disease to others. This forms part of the relational turn that Battin and colleagues impress, in which we are all simultaneously threatening each other in more or less responsible ways. But I think this speaks less to the nature of the interactions the individual has with other individuals, and more to the way their interactions may be (often unjustly) constrained by the society in which they live. Individuals engaging in high-risk behaviors may have a low-wage jobs they rely on for subsistence, or elderly parents that need care, or housing insecurity, or vulnerable immigration status, or simply lack access to healthcare with which they could get medical treatment if they did, in fact, have a disease! These and many other reasons may make someone put themselves in a situation where they expose others to risk in the name of a serious need. Moreover, the nature of public health threats, as I mentioned in chapter 2, are those that individuals are ill-equipped to prepare for alone, and in fact may be penalized in non-pandemic times for doing so.

These individuals, we can say, are *dominated*, meaning their options for acting are restricted on an arbitrary basis.[47] In the above cases, individuals may be implicated in risking the transmission of disease, but their choices are arbitrarily restricted by the kind of society built around them, longstanding historic injustices, and their social mores—even those otherwise encouraged by a society that now demands differently of them.

Dominated individuals aren't nonresponsible threats in the same way as someone innocently shedding virus. But nor are they necessarily liable to defensive harms. To begin, the individuals that might be threatened in these cases may have considerable latitude to avoid a threat—and bear in mind that these dominated individuals are not seeking to harm others but are (1) a component of the causal path through which harm is produced, and (2) placed into a position in this path by virtue of their circumstances. These individuals could plausibly be avoided in many cases or could have the risk they produce reduced in other ways. In this case, their status as vectors is *just* their status as victims. While not the same as the nonresponsible threat in that they strictly speaking have some choice, those choices are extremely limited. Moreover, we may have ways to avoid them entirely, or reduce their risk below the level at which they are a threat to us.[48]

It would be remiss to avoid discussion of individuals who either spread an infectious disease intentionally or who oppose certain kinds of public health measures on spurious grounds. The most obvious and targeted group of these are the unvaccinated. But here, it is not clear that a choice to impose greater risk on others in the event I become a nonresponsible threat is sufficient for me to constitute a threat liable for a defense response. It is certainly wrong of me to increase the chance that I infect someone with a disease if I have an easily available alternative.[49] But that does not necessarily make me more liable for defensive harms just in case I am then put in a circumstance where I unintentionally infect someone. This is like asking why the man falling from the cliff was so close when he fell or was pushed. There is something in the story that made his imposing risk of harm to me more likely, but that does not necessarily generate his liability to be harmed.

In some rare cases, individuals may be liable for defensive harms. The cases I have in mind include, for example, individuals who are aggressive, or act in ways that constitute deliberate acts of disease transmission, such as spitting on people, removing their masks and getting inappropriately close to others, forcibly removing others' masks, and so on. These are individuals that are responsible aggressors. But here, their victim status seems irrelevant. In fact, in legal terms, most of them have already engaged in battery and may be liable in some jurisdictions to self-defensive responses on that alone. But I note that these are very small numbers of cases, much smaller than simple vaccine refusal. Vaccine refusers, in my experience, are often *terrified* of infectious disease, but they have other reasons for imposing risk on the community, rather than being positively interested in causing its spread.

This, then, is the summation of the failure of the patient as victim and vector view. Simply being causally implicated in infectious disease transmission *at the moment of transmission* is not a good measure of our responsibility for that transmission, much less for our liability to be subject to reprisals or liberty-infringing public health measures. The patient as victim and vector, paradoxically, critiques bioethics for its reductive individualism but then resorts to a reductive and individualist conception of public health. Resolving this is an important step in an account of threat in infectious disease. But it can't be done merely through an account of responsibility. Moreover, it can't be done by merely presuming that anyone, at any time, is responsible for disease transmission in a particular way.

An Impersonal Account of Disease

The negative account above shows us how an account of threat posed by humans doesn't quite capture what proponents think when considering threat in public health. A concept of threat might be more useful if we can divorce it from the idea that people are the primary locus of threat to health security. Of course, if and when a biological weapon is used, individuals might be the primary threat—the weaponeers, terrorists, or states that are creating and using a biological weapon. But health security is considerably broader than the issue of biological weapons, and thus examining it in the context of naturally occurring diseases is a first port of call.

The first reason to abandon the anthropocentric view of threat is that, in the broader context of infectious disease, considering humans as the locus of our concern ignores the vast array of nonhuman, non-agential, microbial threats that exist outside of humans *for now*. A central concern of those preparing for and responding to disease pandemics are zoonotic pandemics, those that cross from animals into humans. It seems absurd to imagine that an account of public health threat that only imagines disease becomes a threat when it crosses into humans, any more than it imagines that a forest fire only threatens a town when the first house burns. An account of threat must be broader than that.

Even within humans, imagining humans as threats from the perspective of public health likewise seems mistaken. People are causally implicated in *harm* all the time when we consider infectious disease. The most obvious of these is when we transmit the causative agent of infectious disease to each other. This could be the flu, Ebola virus disease, or a yeast infection. In all of these you are harmed, even if I am unaware I've harmed you. Yet whether I am a threat to you, and that threat arises to make me liable to a defense response, is unclear.

The reasons for that are borne out in related literatures on threat. Consider the unjust combatant hiding among an unwitting group of civilians. Are we permitted to bomb those civilians just in case that combatant is there? Most serious accounts say that on the face of things no, we are not. This is true even if the civilians make it difficult for us to otherwise act against the combatant. Why? Because those civilians, despite unwittingly being causally implicated in some future harm in virtue of shielding the combatant, retain their rights. So too, just because we may unwittingly—say, in asymptomatic cases—play host to a virus does not mean that we lose our rights merely because we are causally implicated for the harms we choose. And importantly, at least in the ethics of armed conflict, this is true even if the civilians are sympathetic to the insurgent, or merely hostile to us.

If involvement in causal stories were sufficient, moreover, we would be permitted to act defensively against all manner of people. It seems plausible, for example, that voting for Ronald Reagan did more to harm US public health through the trajectory of the AIDS crisis alone than any individual currently host to a particular biological pathogen. Even if Reagan voters were not aware that infectious diseases would be the scourge of the twenty-first century, they were still causally responsible for where we are today. But I think people who argue that we should deny people who refuse to get vaccines access to medical insurance would balk at denying Reagan voters (or G. H. W Bush voters, or Clinton voters, or G. W. Bush voters, etc.) access to medical care based on their causal responsibility for pandemic disease.

This is not to deny that individuals may act in a way that increases the risk of transmission of disease. What it poses, however, is a question of how public health actors and policies should regard liability for that risk when choosing actions that infringe on individual rights. And here, the reasons seem thin. Public health policies act on whole communities, sometimes entire nations. If liable threats matter from a normative perspective, they matter at best as secondary considerations; most individuals are either unaware of the risk they pose to others or are in a compromised position by virtue of their arrangement of power in society. And if the response is genuinely necessary, proportionate, and a last resort, liability may be irrelevant: whether an individual is liable to a defensive action just doesn't matter for the purpose of preventing the spread of disease in critical cases.

Here, then, is a case where one can use militarized metaphors in a way that is contrary to mainstream securitized approaches to public health. If healthcare workers are the equivalent to warfighters on the front line, the infected public isn't the equivalent of enemy. The public, rather, is equivalent to noncombatant civilians—even if they are at times hostile or uncooperative civilians, who are absolutely a feature of war. They might be hostages to a disease; they might be human shields. Yes, they sometimes might act in ways that make the enemy's job easier. Some may see the chaos as an opportunity to advance their own ends inside the strife. But they aren't the enemy. What we do in response to their needs, especially when the fate of communities or nations is on the line, is a tricky normative question. But this account of what the public counts transitions us from understanding the public as a threat, much less a threat subject to defensive means by the state, to something requiring considerably stronger moral considerations to target.

Instead, it is the causative agent of disease that is the enemy, and a threat liable to defensive measures. The reference of a non-agential threat may strike some as odd. Rights to self-defense don't inhere in nonsentient beings. I can't exercise my right to self-defense against a toaster unless it is thrown, or dropped, or otherwise used by someone against me. And then my right to self-defense isn't against the toaster, but it's against my attacker. So why should a virus be any different?

This is where we must be careful about what motivates public health, rather than war. War is an exercise of defense of a state against a belligerent: the right of collective self-defense is deeply contested;[50] we typically envisage it against other humans. But we could imagine an armed conflict that mobilized the tools of the state against a non-agent, however. Imagine an army of sophisticated but nonsentient robots, arriving in our solar system with no sentient leader behind them, with simple orders to exterminate humans. Here, I think almost everyone would say that if there is any justification for the use of the armed forces, it is this one! And I think we'd recognize this as war. Even if the use of force is against non-agents, we would still recognize this as some kind of war. It occupies a similar understanding of threat and would require a similar institutional response by states (if not the whole world).

And yet some of the limits of the just war would still apply. Obviously, we can't harm these robots assuming, as we do, that they are not sentient. But war is still hell. If there's some way to prevent the robots from executing their plan without resorting to a catastrophic armed conflict, we should. Not because of the robots, of course: you can't harm a toaster. But you can harm any civilians in theater, and they still matter. This provides both *ad bellum* restrictions, in terms of the decision to mobilize and choose to use that kind of force, and *in bello* in how that force is prosecuted. This is because modern wars are not simply a series of isolated skirmishes but are often industrial affairs that cause harms and violations well beyond the scope of a gun.

The analogy, I take it, is similar. The biological robots called viruses, or their living cousins in other kingdoms,[51] are not sentient. But there is still a case to be made for limits to the kind of force we bring to bear in defending against them, through the institution of public health. In particular, because of the deep costs to humans in mobilizing a public health emergency response, a premium should be placed on avoiding a public health emergency where possible.

This account of public health is homologous, as I noted in the previous chapter, with the basic tenets of just war theory. War is, among other things, a last resort, the option of communities—usually states—when diplomacy has failed. Likewise, public health is, among other things, the task of preventing crises from emerging. Only when we fail does the logic of the health emergency take form. Health security is a departure from routine public health, our analog to peace. But, because of the world as it is, we are justified in preparing for, and thinking through, what happens when we must go to war against disease.

Contingent Pacifism

This impersonal account provides an instrument with which to critically engage public and global health. While we may be justified invoking emergency responses as a last resort, what constitutes a "last resort" is substantially stronger than it appears on its face. Recall that for many, if not most, the threat of disease is either epistemically unavailable to them because they don't or can't know they are infected or, even if they could know, they are unable to respond in a way that protects them and others sufficiently to prevent a global pandemic.

In chapter 2, I introduced the basic idea of contingent pacifism. In the context of armed conflict, Larry May presents contingent pacifism as follows. Traditionally the ethics of armed conflict is cast as a debate between pacifists, who think that no war is ever justified, and realists, who think that war is a normal and indeed permissible extension of state power. Just war theory seeks to find an alternate position of these two views. May argues, however, that rather than just war theory giving us a reason to reject realism, it rather is better positioned historically and normatively to give us a reason to reject pacifism.[52] Contingent pacifism emerges from this inversion to claim not that all wars are unjust, *contra* absolute pacifism: just that all wars that have actually happened, and are likely to happen in the world as it is, are unjust. Part of the reasons for this is that taken seriously, the criteria for declaring war, and then waging it justly, are so demanding the war is almost never necessary, proportionate, a last resort, or pursued for a just cause.[53] Moreover, while wars can be just in one and only one way—a just declaration, just conduct, and just resolution—they can be unjust in many ways.[54] They can be unjustly declared but justly conducted; justly declared and fought but unjustly ended, and so on. Contingent pacifism provides not just a way to specify that wars are frequently if not always unjust in practice but how and why they are unjust, and how the world should change in response to this.

As with war, again, so with public health. Health security's normative foundations, especially in the United States, have largely emerged from what we might consider the equivalent of a realist framework: in armed conflict, the view that war is simply an extension of politics, an inevitable part of the anarchical fabric of international relations. In health security, the realist turn produces scholarship and policy that seek to prevent and respond to disasters but rarely engages substantively with questions of justice within which health emergencies arise.[55] It produces wargame scenarios describing mass casualty events, but—despite acknowledging the fragmented and weak state of American healthcare is likely to be a vulnerability in the nation's defense against infectious disease[56]—it never broaches the question of whether a national health system or insurance would be useful in preventing such a disaster from unfolding.[57] It calls for informing the public about public health actions rapidly,[58] but rarely connects this to larger political issues around the fragmented nature of American public health and marginalized citizens' justified distrust of those systems. And it advocates high science and technology in the form of disease forecasting using real-time health data, among others, but avoids the problem that health data is fragmented and of poor quality precisely because of the commodification of American healthcare.[59] It takes the position, finally, that conflicts between rights are likely and inevitable and seeks to work back from this supposed reality to a position of relative security against communicable diseases.

To restate, health security in practice looks much like a realist school in international relations. Most contemporary health security takes, though never explicitly, the idea that the existing politics of health are simply the ground truth in which it operates, and that this ground truth has no ethical content in and of itself. How states manage health is divorced from how they ought to care about health security.

This position, however, is methodologically backwards and lacking strong, primary moral justification. Rather, an approach that corresponds with contingent pacifism seems a fruitful starting point. This position asserts that health rights, among others, are critical and near inviolable. These rights extend broadly from individual medical care out to international (even global) health governance. They are, moreover, inseparable from broader political, social, economic, and social rights. Needing to make trade-offs of the kind that health security and the orthodox position envisions, is in principle possible but in practice is rarely inevitable or necessary and may never even be just in the real world. It should only be taken as a last resort, when our ability to negotiate with ourselves and with our natural environment has broken down.

We don't need to be what I consider to be the public health equivalent of a pacifist, or what Gostin accuses individuals such as Annas of in his comments on "left libertarians." But we can accept that, as a critical move, no public health emergency has or could be just in the world in which we live, because none took the threat of the causal agent of disease, and the lack of liability of individuals, seriously: evidenced alone by decades of repeat, unheeded calls that we are "not ready for the next pandemic."[60] This doesn't discount that public health emergency actions may be required to respond to the threat of disease. But even if we are forced to act this way, we might not satisfy the demands of just health security.

Ecology

If the causative agent of disease is the enemy, then where the enemy comes from matters. Particularly in a securitized public health setting, the idea that communicable disease threatens a community is central to justifying the defense of communities in public health. As this is a book about public health crises, a central question is where likely pandemic diseases will emerge.

Where the rubber hits the road is in creating the conditions that cause pandemics to arise. Not all pandemics have their origins in human affairs, but many do. The emergence of coronaviruses as zoonotic pandemic pathogens has been linked to encroachments on the natural habitats of bats and other intermediate species.[61] Flu is primarily an avian disease, but increasing interaction between displaced wild bird populations and domestic fowl or pigs creates the opportunity for spillover events.[62] Likewise, the deforestation caused by heavy industry in sub-Saharan Africa drives the emergence of Ebola virus disease.[63]

The density of pathogens is linked closely, moreover, to biodiversity. The most biodiverse areas on the planet, however, have long histories of colonization and resource exploitation that have seriously, and perhaps irrevocably, damaged these landscapes. Our obligations to prevent public health emergency are shaped, on a basic level, by the background institutions of nations and indeed the global community.

Climate change renders all this more extreme. The emergence of Zika virus as a public health emergency of international concern in Latin America has been tied to the increasing ranges of the *Aedes* mosquito, which transmits Zika but also Yellow Fever and other deadly diseases. As the globe warms from anthropogenic climate change, these host ranges are projected to change further, driving increasing numbers of pandemics.[64]

A contingent pacifist position of public health holds, as its analogue in just war, that the use of force to manage a public health crisis is justified only as a last resort. This is because the emergency responses we have seen in the context of COVID-19 are only justified when we have done what we can to prevent needing to declare an emergency. Yet it is hard to see how we are anywhere close to that last resort, given the current international approach to climate change and the ongoing and systemic deprivations in our world. Take the 2013–2016 Ebola outbreak, credited sometimes as a disease brought about by "bushmeat."[65] Yet a closer examination of the crisis shows that outbreak was brought about, in no small part, by the legacy of colonialism and civil war, and exploitative industrial practices by developed nations in Western Africa that left the three target countries unable to defend themselves, through conventional public health, from the virus.[66] This is not a claim against the nations of Liberia, Sierra Leone, and Guinea, but rather a claim against the nations who, over the last hundred years, have systematically deprived these nations of their ability to withstand a disease epidemic of this kind. The most recent outbreak of Ebola virus disease in Kivu province of the Democratic Republic of the Congo, similarly, arose in part because of ongoing civil conflict borne of Belgian colonization.[67] COVID-19 has been likewise credited, among other things, as a product of global trends toward insular responses, away from global solidarity, and away from robust public health.[68]

In all these cases, to paraphrase a famous thought experiment by David Mitchell and Robert Webb, we are the bad guys.[69] The impersonal account of disease pits us against the causative agent of disease, yes. But any serious look at the actions of humans on this planet identifies us as *a*, if not *the*, belligerent party in many if not most of these conflicts. Infectious disease is indeed terrible, but it is as much a consequence of human interference with natural environments as it is anything else.

This is not, of course, to say that humans must ultimately bear the fate of infectious disease.[70] Rather, the liability resides with states individually and jointly to invest in mechanisms that prevent the need for public health emergency responses. Climate change mitigation, then, is not only a justified public health measure; it is *obligatory* just in case it presents a tractable and less coercive alternative to another public health crisis like COVID-19. Likewise, policies that allow initially symptomatic individuals to report their symptoms, undergo isolation and care without fear of reprisals or domination, are not just desirable but obligatory just in case it prevents the seeding of a global pandemic. It arguably unites the twin tasks of universal health coverage and health security. It is not enough to have a strong medical system, vaccines, and medical countermeasures to pathogens of concern. Rather, individuals need to be able to access that health system with relative confidence in their treatment and outcomes in order to prevent a health emergency from arising.

This provides us with, in philosophical terms, a compelling ideal theory. It does not abandon the basic tenets of health security, but nor does it grant them a starting position akin to political realism. Rather, it takes as its starting point the view that communicable disease pandemics are indeed a true threat to humans and their communities. It inverts this, however, to say that because of the source of that threat, and the people that are harmed in the process of mobilizing state power in emergent contexts, we should avoid the conflict where possible.

Objections and Complications

An easy response to all of this is as follows. Sure, the impersonal account of disease is desirable. But, if we are going to combat infectious disease, we have to account for the actions of individuals and groups that either deliberately spread disease or take actions they know or should reasonably expect to cause the transmission of infectious disease. Sometimes, individuals are complicit in the spread of disease, and on a mass scale. We might note observations of the outsized role that "superspreading events" play in the transmission of COVID-19 as evidence that particular individuals are responsible for a large number of cases.[71]

The term "super spreader" has its own terrible history that I will not get into here, and perhaps there is partial victory in the assignment of that phrase to events and no longer people.[72] To address this let's set aside first the role of congregate settings in super spreading events, as these fall neatly into my previous analysis. The US meat industry, or prison system, are both settings of horrific injustices that coerce and dominate individuals, and their responsibility in super spreading events is a nonstarter. For those that are left, the question then becomes twofold, between principles and policies.

I maintain that even with this remainder, there remains an open question about the degree to which individuals are responsible for something like a super-spreader event. The first part of that question is simply empirical, and it goes back to the HIV/AIDS crisis. The original "patient zero," Gaëten Dugas, was considered for a long time to be the origin of the disease in the United States, until later studies confirmed that he was one of only many early cases in the 1970s.[73] So there are frequently empirical uncertainties in establishing that someone is responsible for spreading disease, much less that they are responsible for a particular cluster. And, given that most individuals are not liable to a defensive response, we should hold our priors strongly against being able to identify such individuals and refrain from unjustly harming them.[74]

But beyond this, I suspect, as above, that the actual degree to which we can hold individuals responsible is simply suspect. Very few nations adopt not just as social mores but as institutional and organizational policy that if you are sick, you should stay home. The United States is a nation in which going to work, or even just out into public sick is not only expected—it is socially enforced through a web of esteem. One study found that 38 percent of Americans admit to working while sick, and the overwhelming majority of those work while infected with a respiratory virus.[75] This is undoubtedly different in countries with more robust social welfare systems, but paid time off among other support systems to encourage individuals to socially distance is highly heterogeneous worldwide. We should ask carefully, then, the degree to which we have set up a society where we really take the idea that people are responsible for transmitting infectious disease seriously, given we routinely tell them they should risk others as a matter of course. This looks more like a social system of risk sharing: and if that is true but also undesirable, we are obligated to change the system of sharing rather than punish people for it.

A second foreseeable objection is the degree to which this account of the impersonal account of disease is compatible with the rest of public health. Even if we accepted this account for communicable diseases and pandemics in particular, there is a general predisposition in public health toward identifying the behavioral causes of diseases. This is perhaps best summed up in McGinnis and Foege's "Actual Causes of Death in the United States," which in 1993 identified individual behavioral traits—smoking status, dietary choices, activity, and alcohol—as the "actual" contributors to mortality in the United States.[76]

This is an old debate in public health and there is not sufficient time to cover it all. McGinnis and Foege's analysis is by their admission driven partly by the factors they can quantify; the ability to measure something, however, is not evidence that it is the relevant cause of that thing. The pair do acknowledge the "Whitehall study" of British civil servants that identified a relationship between salary and incidence of coronary heart disease, commonly seen as the progenitor of the "social determinants of health" movement.[77] These divergences point to a large normative issue in American public health, and insofar as the impersonal account of disease is anything, it is an extension of that larger debate that falls squarely into the latter camp. And while the impersonal account of disease is primarily positioned to account for health security concerns, it can give a normative account of why McGinnis and Foege, and indeed other writers, are wrong to identify diet or other "actual" cause of disease as the product of mere individual choice. That account is of domination—dietary behaviors, among others, are strongly moderated by access to food, ability to purchase, and time to prepare, all of which are determined by the social factors that arbitrarily restrict people's choices.[78] This isn't to discount the autonomy of individuals, as domination is a political philosophical account of freedom rather than an individual normative capacity like autonomy.[79] Rather, the impersonal account of disease says about noncommunicable diseases the same as it does communicable diseases: there is little justification, and little truth, in considering individuals as threats to the public in view of their disease state that justifies a defensive response. As I will discuss in the next chapter, there may even be reasons where there is broad societal agreement that some states of ill-health are not only permissible, but that society ought to support through public health and health care regardless.

A final concern is that there may be a segment of society that is, in effect, helping the enemy—that is, individuals who are either intentionally helping the spread of disease or are acting in such a way that the spread of disease furthers their instrumental goals. Here, too, the war metaphor can help us. It may be that sometimes we perform acts that infringe on civilian rights when those civilians pose an operational risk to a justified war. However, again the concern about intentionality is perhaps important only in terms of the proportionality if we assume that intention tracks effectiveness in some way. Whether individuals compromise an operation accidentally (by shouting in exclamation because they are surprised) or intentionally (to alert the enemy) is beside the point. The question is whether there is proportionate reason to infringe on their rights to prevent some other harm and achieve a necessary aim to end a crisis.[80]

There may be a time, however, when officials, or personnel, are guilty of something like *perfidy*, the crime of wearing the colors of allies when one is an enemy. That is, they might be able to help with response to a pandemic, or preventing a pandemic, but ultimately and intentionally decide to act in a way that knowingly causes death by infectious disease when they are tasked with protecting people against a pandemic. This is a serious charge, and how it fits into health security requires a deeper interrogation into the roles of officials in a public health institution. But two things are worth noting here. The first is that similar to distinctions in war, what it means for members of an armed forces unit to commit wrongdoing is professionally linked to the powers they have to achieve their goals. So committing wrongdoing as professionals is significantly more morally weighty than committing wrongdoing by noncombatants, even if that wrongdoing is quite serious. But the second, and more important clarification is that what it means to hold those professionals accountable, and how we do so, is a contested area. Punitive measures may be insufficient in cases of mass harm, and restorative measures such as truth and reconciliation commissions may be more appropriate. How we resolve this is beyond the scope of this book. But I note we are less likely to be able to plausibly accuse a neighbor of perfidy for refusing to mask, than we are a senator who uses knowledge of the pandemic to alter policy for financial gain.

Conclusion

In this chapter I established the impersonal account of the threat of disease: one in which the appropriate referent of a health security threat is, in the case of naturally arising diseases, the causative agent of communicable disease. I showed how this connected to larger analogues to the ethics of war, and how the disruption of a health emergency establishes a last resort clause in the deflation of health emergency. This last resort clause, I concluded, was strong enough that it established strong obligations to prevent the contexts that lead to pandemics, including the environmental, national structural, and international political contexts that create the conditions in which pandemics thrive and require limits on liberty.

In the next chapter, we can complete an account of the ethics of declaring a public health emergency by addressing health emergencies directly. Having completed an account of the public health state, and the appropriate threat against which it can be mobilized in liberty-limiting ways, we can now establish a set of criteria for justly declaring a public health emergency.

5 The Moral Foundations of the Public Health State

War is, in the main, an act carried out by communities. In the modern era, one constant in war[1] is the presence of at least one nation-state.[2] Wars may be fought between nation-states, within nation-states, or by outside groups against nation-states. In all of these, however, the state plays a role.

So, too, with public health. At the highest level, authority for public health stems from the state. Medicine is the practice of protecting and healing individuals. Public health is the social control of the conditions that lead to the development and spread of disease; it inheres to communities. Hodge Jr. and Gostin go far enough to say that "protecting public health during an emergency is an essential goal of government."[3]

The role of the state is most obvious when the subject of public health is communicable disease. A critical step in securitizing disease, historically, is the recognition that infectious diseases "don't respect borders." The IHR exist, among other things, as an agreement between states to report disease outbreaks that may be a threat to the global community, and to coordinate and act to prevent the spread of infectious disease.[4] As such, the nation-state becomes, at least right now, a critical actor in preventing the transmission of disease, in virtue of its ability to maintain borders and enforce restrictions on the movements of people and goods across the world.

In chapter 3, I noted that a central historical connection between public health ethics and military ethics was Childress's account of the just war as grounded in legitimate authority. I argued this connection was not necessary to motivate the connection between military and public health ethics, and that it was better to formulate health security as a response to threat. I provided that formulation in the last chapter. But discussions of legitimacy are essential to justifying the role of public health as an *institution* with moral ends, and to the use of force by the state to achieve those ends. By institution, I mean a part of general social arrangements, laws, norms, and political entities that provide for an important dimension of social and political life. National security, I have argued, is an institution,[5] and public health is if not its own institution, a major component of the broader institution of health.[6]

In the previous chapter I argued that a key issue for health security has been its tendency to flatten public health concerns and favor technocratic solutions that, for example, deprioritize basic public health while overemphasizing the creation of novel therapeutics.[7] One reason for this, I articulated, is that health security appeals to what is presumed to be the common and nonpartisan appeal of national security to advance its aims. Dazak did this, recall, in appealing to, of all things, the war on terror to motivate stronger public health. National security, I suspect, is presumed by health security to be "apolitical" in that its status quo existence is agreed to by a broad segment of society. What could argue against the need for national self-defense?

This move has largely been a failure, if the nature of global health governance is anything to go by. This is partly because national security is not "apolitical." In particular—as a widespread global phenomenon—national security frequently receives widespread support when it concerns buying of new hardware, but not when it comes to expanding the diplomatic corps, providing humanitarian aid to stabilize regions, and developing strategic relationships that are mutually beneficial to all parties for the purpose of common advancement. National security is "apolitical" only if it is conservative, hawkish, and militaristic, and even then I suspect only because there are social mechanisms to maintain that group dynamic in the national security community. To borrow from the literature on the politics of governance, national security has been depoliticized, placed at a remove from the contested nature of politics and governance, quite intentionally.[8] But doing so has been the product of a series of specific policy and political choices.

A considerable amount of research has documented the turmoil as civil society has tried to offer an alternative to this current state of affairs and I won't rehash that history here.[9] Rather, what is important is that the substantive moral foundations of the national security state are not the subject of a broad consensus, and perhaps not a consensus at all. Assuming so as a foundation for health security, and public health more broadly, is thus a mistake. And while I claimed there is a homology between public health ethics and just war theory, a robust account of the *public health state* is needed to establish just why that is.

In what follows, I tie the aims of public health to the state and ground the state as the legitimate authority in public health. But I do so in a way that sets up the problem of what Michael Moehler has called "deep pluralism," and the limits on what a rational but divided people can accept for public health. I begin with justifications for public health as a state institution with which many will be familiar: libertarianism, contract theories in the liberal tradition, and utilitarianism. I show how each gives us an account of public health as a state institution, but one that clashes deeply with other commitments of members of states, and over which conflicts will need to be resolved.

I argue that most theories of public health ethics do not provide a robust means for thinking through what could justify a robust public health state—including health security's place in that state—that can account for deep pluralism. Given the deep tensions in modern states, and the currently unsubstantiated assumption by health security researchers and practitioners about shared values, it is appropriate to motivate a view of public health that can be sensitive to the need to resolve conflicts between individual agents. Moreover, this view gives us an account of political philosophy that justifies a very robust public health institution.

Public Health and Legitimacy

The question of legitimacy is critical to public health which, while often local in its ultimate practice, is still a broad collective enterprise. As a collective enterprise, we require an account of how we establish rules, enforce them, and represent the interests of individuals engaged in the enterprise in a way they can endorse. Importantly, legitimacy is a key component of modern claims against the state interfering with, or neglecting, the health of marginalized communities. This is particularly important in the domain of health. To take an example from outside mainstream health security, in his book on disability rights, James Charlton notes in his introduction to activism by the disability community:

> For the first time in recorded human history politically active people with disabilities are beginning to proclaim that they know what is best for themselves and their community. This is a militant, revelational claim aptly capsulized in "Nothing About Us Without Us."[10]

This famous saying, "nothing about us without us," is reflected in the struggle for recognition and treatment by the state in HIV/AIDS activist communities. In his *How to Survive a Plague*, David France describes the May 21, 1990, protest at the NIH headquarters to demand that the AIDS community play a guiding role in coordinating the national effort to end the epidemic. After an incident involving violence against a protestor, a press conference was held in which Dr. Anthony Fauci—who would become a hero of the COVID-19 epidemic thirty years later—claimed the protest was "interesting theater. But it was not helpful." Keith Cylar responded:

> I think Fauci understands, and at times appreciates, what we do. Fauci himself understands that he does not have the power himself to do what needs to be done. That's why the system has to open up.[11]

A critical demand of ACT UP was that government excluded individuals with HIV/AIDS from determining how and when their needs would be met, and how an epidemic that involved them would be managed. His comment on Fauci is instructive as a comment on the limits of civil service—the National Institutes of Health in the United States is a part of the executive branch of government—to accomplish just goals through their own means. In both this and the case of disability, the implicit message is this: the state is only legitimate insofar as it is a reflection of, and promotes, an appropriate set of interests of its citizenry. It must be responsive to those interests in order to be legitimate.

The public health ethics theories canvased in chapter 3 assume a certain structure of or legitimacy of public health and/or health security, namely the existence of a broad agreement as to the values, norms, and institutions of the (usually American) state. I want to start to take the opposite tack. Thomas Hobbes, famously, gives us a thought experiment in the form of the state of nature, a world without government, in which all humans war against all others for survival. As a key move in his political philosophy, Hobbes notes that in this world, human options are extremely constrained:

> Whatsoever therefore is consequent to a time of Warre, where every man is Enemy to every man; the same is consequent to the time, wherein men live without other security, than what their own strength, and their own invention shall furnish them withall. In such condition, there is no place for Industry; because the fruit thereof is uncertain; and consequently no Culture of the Earth; no Navigation, nor use of the commodities that may be imported by Sea; no commodious Building; no Instruments of moving, and removing such things as require much

force; no Knowledge of the face of the Earth; no account of Time; no Arts; no Letters; no Society; and which is worst of all, continuall feare, and danger of violent death; And the life of man, solitary, poore, nasty, brutish, and short.[12]

This ties the security of the state to human endeavor. Moreover, I think it captures something about pandemic disease, and certainly COVID-19 bears some of this out. Being unable to interact with each other for fear of a threat (even if nonresponsible, as I argued in the previous chapter) undermines more than simply our health in the case of infection. It alters life plans in serious ways, stalling careers (or in the case of young people preventing them from beginning); ends personal relationships or prevents them from flourishing; generates new economic injustices or exacerbates the old; disables trade and commerce; undermines the pursuit of knowledge; and leaves us in a state of constant fear of death.

While the state of nature is a philosophical tool, it is on its face a good analog to the disordered world in which public health does not govern the health of communities, or does not exist—close to the world we live in today. This is a world without any health security: indeed, the state of nature is a world that is absent security.[13] The justification for effective public health is then simply the observation that no rational person wants to live like this, and the state provides a mechanism for community health to be regulated, including the long-term and even intergenerational effects of illness in communities, as a way to escape this state of nature. What the details of this look like, however, is a harder question.

This is the realm of political philosophy, rather than ethics. Bioethics has not spent much time on political philosophy, or on questions of how the states and political communities ought to be structured. But these questions are essential insofar as public health is a political institution. Three basic justifications for public health often mentioned are libertarianism, liberal egalitarianism typically represented by liberal contract theories, and utilitarianism.[14] These are less concretely theories so much as *families* of theories, with considerable variation within each family, so I sketch these primarily for readers who are not familiar with them.

Libertarianism

Libertarianism holds that rights govern all transactions between individuals, and that almost all other nonconsenting transfers are coercive and illegitimate. Robert Nozick, arguably one of the more famous proponents of this theory, establishes a hypothetical society in which there exists a "just set of initial acquisitions," some just arrangement of goods in the world. All individuals have a set of rights to life and property and may be deprived of those goods only under conditions of contract, for example, consenting transfers between individuals. All other transfers are illegitimate and coercive, and famously libertarians consider progressive taxation as "coercive" in this sense.[15]

Typically, the sole exception to this is the so-called night-watchman state, which justifies a modicum of national security that may require taxation to stand up. The basic justification here is that all individuals in a particular community have a right to defend themselves, but no one person can accomplish this against either internal (criminal) or external (military) threats. This coordination problem, and the seriousness of these infractions in that one cannot be compensated for one's death (among other things) by contract, sets up a justification for a national security apparatus that the state may fund.

Nozick's views (and, I suspect, other libertarian views) are almost certainly incoherent on their own grounds.[16] On the one hand, no such set of just initial acquisitions exists in practice, and would presumably require considerable redistributive transfers to rectify.[17] On the other, the precise contours of why the night watchman state can be motivated but no other public service, are opaque. But Nozick does provide the most plausible version of libertarianism and has made what I consider a good-faith rational reconstruction of his views.

In terms of public health, we could imagine a similar justification to the night watchman state: a "night nurse state." That is, individuals have rights to life and property, but are sometimes unable to adequately coordinate against internal (locally transmitted) or external (pandemic) threats. Some analogue to the night watchman state, but for public health, might be justified to coordinate against these threats to individual rights.

Note, however, that this is still a very, *very* thin account of public health. It would provide no rationale for most public health surveillance, health programs, antismoking campaigns, disability insurance, health insurance, data or sample sharing, foreign aid, threat reduction programs, capacity building in other nations, childhood vaccination programs, nutrition programs, and so on. Of note, where in a previous chapter I charged Gostin with conflating libertarianism and liberalism (which he contrasts together with communitarianism), this is one important separation between liberal and libertarian theories. Libertarian theories offer almost nothing in the way of a state beyond merely enforcing contracts and protecting life in very specific ways.

At best, a night nurse state would likely concentrate only on communicable diseases that

1. are transmitted without the knowledge of the carrier;
2. spread fast enough and are deadly enough that containing them is both in the interest of all community members because it threatens their ability to form any reliable contracts or maintain the minimal state, but is not able to be accomplished via individual coordination.

This is obviously a very small set of public health concerns. But note here that this restrictiveness does not pertain to rights themselves, but to the particular architecture of rights that holds them to be inviolable and justifies only minimal state involvement. Someone like Nozick, I suspect, would hold that it might be *good*, all things considered, if people didn't die from smoking that was causally implicated to predatory advertising campaigns. But he would likewise maintain that there is no justification for the state to intervene in consenting parties doing that to themselves—and likewise, no justification for the use of taxation to fund a health insurance system that would care for those people if they do develop lung cancer caused by smoking. Likewise, so long as it does not disrupt the state and the ability to make contracts, he would oppose most pandemic responses on the grounds that individual rights to choose and contract on their own terms are more important than even thousands, or hundreds of thousands of deaths.

Liberal Contract Theories

It is likely that just as libertarianism gives us a minimal "night watchman" security state, it will also give us no more than a minimal "night nurse" approach to public health providing protection from the worst public health crises, but not much else. This limitation is in part why Gostin's conflation of liberalism and libertarianism is egregious: the view they give us of the justification of public health, and thus the moral limits of the use of power or force by public health institutions (the idiosyncrasies of what libertarians consider "force" aside), are divergent.

There are a range of alternatives available, the largest group of which I'll simply refer to as contract theories. There are quite a number of flavors of these theories in contemporary political philosophy, and some of them have received attention in public health ethics.[18] However, I will stick with arguably the most influential of these theories on the field, Rawls's theory of justice spanning forty years of the twentieth and twenty-first centuries. His central theory, justice as fairness, was presented in *Theory of Justice*; I will draw from *Theory*, but also from his later *Justice as Fairness: A Restatement*, which serves to clarify Rawls's work at the end of his life.

Rawls's theory of justice as fairness emerges as a response to utilitarian political philosophy (see below), drawn from Kantian claims that—very loosely put—we should respect the interests and agency of individual persons. Rawls argues that to establish principles of justice, we should imagine rationally self-interested agents discussing the creation of an ideal society. These agents are in the *original position* and must all agree on the circumstances of justice. They are, moreover, under a *veil of ignorance* where they do not know the circumstances under which they will live in this society, including class, gender, race, natural abilities, and so on.[19] The original position under the veil of ignorance is justified by Rawls as a precondition for fair and equal negotiations between parties in establishing the basis of fair cooperation. The original position allows citizens to reach, for themselves, an agreement that is fair for all. The veil of ignorance, according to Rawls, is one in which negotiating citizens have a point of view that is not distorted by the particular features and circumstances of the existing basic structure of society.[20]

The result, Rawls claims, is a form of risk aversion that arrives at two principles of justice:

1. Each person has the same indefeasibility claim to a fully adequate scheme of equal basic liberties, which scheme is compatible with the same scheme of liberties for all; and

2. Social and economic inequalities are to satisfy two conditions: first, they are to be attached to offices and position open to all under conditions of fair equality of opportunity; and second, they are to be to the greatest benefit of the least-advantaged members of society (the difference principle).[21]

Rawls has received sustained criticism of his treatment, or lack thereof, of features including race,[22] gender, and the family structure,[23] and health and disability as instantiations of justice or relevant features in formulating a just society.[24] The most important one for our purposes is the last, and Norman Daniels extends Rawls by identifying what he considers to be a critical component of Rawls's theory: protecting the opportunities of citizens, both as a condition of realizing the first principle of justice and as an explicit part of the difference principle. It follows, Daniels argues, that if promoting health helps to protect opportunity, then meeting health needs protects opportunity. Since Rawls requires us to protect opportunity, it follows that Rawls also requires us to protect health, especially as part of the difference principle.[25]

Daniels's work does not explicitly deal with the legitimacy of the public health state, but his work provides a guide. On the one hand, the original position behind the veil of ignorance provides us no information about our health states, or future health states over time, in society. Rational agents engaged in justifying the basic structure of society will thus support, through the difference principle, a basic structure that is expected to protect their opportunities whatever they might be. Agents would thus support a state that administers public health insofar as it protects those opportunities and maximizes the welfare of the worst off.

This kind of state is distinct from the libertarian state partly because it authorizes transfers to fund a public health state that satisfies the difference principle. Moreover, basic liberties are justified as claims against state interference only insofar as they are coextensive with everyone else's liberty. Presumably, this means that the state has some quarantine power—it may restrict movement of individuals or goods that pose a risk to the lives of others, contingent on those restrictions being in principle equally applied across the population. It may also legislate against a broad array of market failures if they benefit the worst off. These include things like occupational and environmental harms, fraudulent manufacture of medical goods, cost of pharmaceuticals, infection control, and so on.

This account, however, doesn't necessarily establish public health as a central feature of the state. Much of what we care about in health—and public health in particular— may be derived from the more general right to life, but only insofar as they are connected either to the violation of that right, or to the effect pursuit of an individual's ends.[26] It is unlikely an independent, *positive* right to health exists under a Rawlsian scheme, such as might justify access and benefit-sharing schemes to pharmaceuticals outside traditional markets, or access to universal healthcare beyond the scope of protecting some minimal set of opportunities, or equitable vaccine distribution.

Rawls noted in later work that he took the basic liberties to be essentially negative in their conception, and that any positive elements were derivable from the background conditions of a property-owning democracy, together with fair equality of opportunity and the difference principle.[27] This is why, coupled with the difference principle, Battin and colleagues' account of Rawls leading to solidarity-based approaches to public health is mistaken. Improving the worst-off representative group in society is not the same as improving the worst situation for every person in that society, nor is solidarity captured under a scheme of basic liberties. Rather, liberalism under Rawls is a modification to the status quo of capitalism in a democracy much like the United States.

Rawls's work assumes that the difference principle does not significantly trade off equality for utility. However, this may not always be so in the case of health. Selgelid gives us an example of an anencephalic child—born with no brain above the brain stem—that can be kept alive for a long time but only through the use of immense amounts of resources. If we assume some level of scarcity, and that being born with anencephaly makes one relatively "the worst off," then the difference principle may mandate allocation of resources to these children at the expense of potentially many, many other needy people who are only slightly better off but can have their situation improved with the application of comparatively fewer resources.[28]

Utilitarianism

A utilitarian public health state would start from a general consequentialist framework of:

1. Some theory of what constitutes a good state of affairs;
2. A way to rank different states of affairs;
3. A way to select between states of affairs as a guide to what one ought to do.

Act utilitarianism's account of these three elements is that a good state of affairs is identified in terms of its pleasure and/or pain, satisfaction of individual preferences, or some objective list of goods (i.e., utility); that one state of affairs is better than another just in case the probability-adjusted sum of all utilities in the former is greater than the latter (aggregation); and that the selection method is just the act of ranking states of affairs. Utilitarianism has experienced a recent resurgence in health security circles with interest in the Effect Altruist movement in global catastrophic biological risks.[29]

A starting point in thinking about public health is what utilitarianism can and can't do about healthcare. Allen Buchanan argues that utilitarianism is incapable of providing a universal right to a decent minimum of healthcare.[30] As with any concern for rights for utilitarianism, it cannot in principle guarantee *anything* to people, but is always contingent on promoting the greatest aggregate utility. It may be, as Buchanan notes, that there is some possible world in which access to healthcare as a matter of rights does in fact promote the greatest utility, but Buchanan claims that under a plausible conception of the actual world we live in, a universal right to healthcare would not in fact do so.

However, public health and access to healthcare is not the same, and here utilitarianism is much simpler and easier than the previous two positions I've discussed in establishing the public health state. First, if we take health as a component of,[31] or precondition to achieving well-being,[32] we ought to promote public health just in case it promotes aggregate well-being in a population. And on this count, famous public health policies do so very straightforwardly: the Salk vaccine, smallpox eradication, and fluoridation are unequivocal successes that have raised up the health of millions of people around the world, and delivered us—in the case of the second—a world free of a microbial scourge.

Second, a utilitarian public health state relates strongly to contemporary health security. The emergence of "global catastrophic risks," risks that threaten the continuity of meaningful human society,[33] as a field of study and policy activism dovetails with the post-2001 concern about bioterrorism and genetically modified viruses with pandemic potential as a rationale for public health. Measures that could prevent the onset of a catastrophic risk (of biological origin or otherwise) could save billions of actual lives, and moreover benefits potential *trillions* of future lives by maintaining a human community that can eventually become spacefaring and expand into the rest of the universe.[34] Very little of the catastrophic risk literature does anything so prosaic as advocate basic public health. One reason I have been given by a member of this community is that catastrophic risks will largely be of an exigency that preventing them is almost always the only way to survive them—health systems cannot, in any real sense, be prepared for them. But in almost all subcatastrophic but still devastating events, public health is worthwhile and desirable.

Three more things should be said about this basic justification. First, utilitarianism is agnostic about the state as the locus of public health. If the nation-state is the entity best poised to maximize utility, utilitarianism recognizes it. But subnational or supranational mechanisms may be better equipped or more likely to maximize expected utility. I set this aside for now; as long as there are still states, utilitarianism can recognize their role as coordinating actors, and I suspect a public health move that seeks to disband the state is likely seen as intractable by most contemporary utilitarians.

Second, utilitarian appeals to public health will likely be *radically* agnostic about public health as an institution. It is unconcerned about what "counts" as public health, and only with promoting expected aggregate utility. So if labor rights promote public health as a means to promoting global utility, then utilitarians should care about labor rights. Utilitarians, I suspect, must care about public health, but will be—to health security and public health practitioners, maddeningly so—unconcerned about the form that takes.

Finally, unlike libertarian and liberal egalitarian accounts, utilitarians have a much less complicated approach to liberty-limiting measures. On criminalization and other punitive public health measures, utilitarians only care about guilt, praise and blame, or responsibility, if those concepts promote expected aggregate utility. It is empirically unlikely they do in most cases. But conversely, utilitarians are also likely to be unconcerned about liberty-limiting public health measures, no matter how coercive, just so long as they promote expected utility. So, utilitarians are not in principle opposed to quarantining or even killing the sick to protect the public. They may have empirical reasons to suggest why this is not the best option to pursue, but nothing in act utilitarianism itself means these are in principle impermissible.

Utilitarianism nonetheless has an important role in liberal thought about public health through John Stuart Mill's "harm principle." In his *On Liberty*, Mill claims "The only purpose for which power can be rightfully exercised over any member of a civilized community, against his will, is to prevent harm to others."[35] While *On Liberty* is subordinate to Mill's utilitarianism,[36] the harm principle[37] is a mainstay of liberal thought and, even when not explicitly identified with utilitarian work, is its most enduring contribution.[38]

Problems of Deep Pluralism

A central problem we arrive at is that these accounts diverge in their account of legitimacy in a public health state, and in the limits and powers such a state ought to have. Accounting for why we should grant the public health state legitimacy is thus deeply contested. This is a problem for a public health state that seeks to justify *publicly* its legitimacy and the powers it has, and is, I suspect, partly what justifies the good-faith turn to national security as "apolitical."

By "deeply pluralistic" I mean that justifications for the public health state are justifications that exist in a world in which the basic tenets of liberalism are not preserved even within ostensibly liberal nations. It is a world inhabited, and in which we must appeal to liberal agents, nonliberal agents, and nonmoral agents alike.[39] Given that public health ethics is, like the rest of bioethics, a discipline ultimately grounded in philosophical justifications for practical actions, we should take this deep pluralism seriously.

Previous attempts to accommodate this pluralism run into trouble. The work of Childress and colleagues—or, at least, the connection between Childress's earlier work and "Mapping the Terrain"—represents what some call mid-level theorizing.[40] That is, the authors take that a particular set of duties or considerations arise intuitively, are noninclusive and subject to revision and/or trade-offs in particular contexts. They are, however, subject to agreement in liberal, secular societies of the kind they envisage, like the US. This is broadly consistent with the position of bioethical principlism made famous by Childress and Tom Beauchamp.[41] I suspect as well that it broadly aligns with Moreno's position on American pragmatism in bioethics, where "actual moral problems are living problems and problems of living; they are 'contested' or embedded in states of affairs,"[42] Kass's procedural approach described in chapter 3, and Gostin's general claims around liberalism.

An alternate strategy is one advocated by Michael Selgelid, concerning "moderating values." This strategy holds that central values promoted by libertarianism, liberal theories, and utiltiarianism—liberty, equality, and utility, respectively—are all fundamentally valuable. The major shortcoming in each theory, then, is not that it fails to signal some important value but that it takes a single value to be either the only important value, or the most important of a ranked list of values. Selgelid, instead, suggests these values "moderate" one another. In some cases, utility will outweigh liberty and equality; in others, liberty will outweigh utility and equality; and in some, equality will outweigh liberty and utility. No one value is more important than another. Selgelid claims finally that there remains, then, some empirical question about when each value is or is not important, and in what way.[43]

Both approaches, however, struggle with deep pluralism. Mid-level theorizing relies heavily on social context; it does not give us a reason to establish public health in either (1) a national context in which there are significant segments of the population who cannot agree on what general moral commitments we ought to have, much less which one is important when; or (2) when we are required to engage in deliberation between those in the local context the mid-level theory derives from, and agents from elsewhere. This, it seems, is a consistent problem for approaches in bioethics and public health ethics broadly that assume a very particular view of the United States (or, more charitably, the Anglophone world) as a starting point when our concerns—as with many public health crises—are so much larger. These theories might conceivably work in practice in clinical scenarios where the number of actors and their views is somewhat limited but fall apart (as any theory would) when its assumptions no longer hold. A sociologist might have more to say on *why* this very particular group of mostly white, mostly elite scholars would have such a view of America, and how they might struggle to explain public health ethics in a country that has a long, history of deep moral divisions, but this is not that kind work.

Moderating values approaches fail, in a similar fashion, just in case we can't agree on which set of values is fundamental, or where there is substantial disagreement about which value is outweighed by another in a broad range of cases. This could be because of framing issues: one way to solve the anencephalic child case, for example, is to claim that the fault lies not with Rawls or with the demands of justice, but with the system that requires a child to die when we could redeploy significant resources from national defense, or policing, or increase marginal taxation rates, and so on. But in other cases, we may simply have incredibly divergent views on what matters. In either case we are stuck with deep pluralism.

Minimal Morality and the Public Health State

Because public health is at least in part a political philosophical problem, novel strategies exist within that literature to accommodate the problem of deep pluralism. The one I shall develop arises from Michael Moehler's work in his *Minimal Morality*.[44] Moehler develops an account of political theory that arises from a minimal conception of human commitments beyond pure instrumental reason. Moehler asks what individuals could agree to if they were

1. forward-looking; that is, capable of having interests in the future;
2. instrumentally rational; that is, capable of adopting suitable means to their ends;
3. self-interested; that is, privilege their own interests ahead of those of others except in cases where it is mutually advantageous to do otherwise;
4. conflict resolving, which Moehler specifies as possessing the "overriding goal of securing peaceful long-term cooperation."

In this minimal level of morality, Moehler claims, solutions to political-philosophical problems can be described as ones that can be endorsed by agents that satisfy only the above conditions. Moehler has defended not just a democratic welfare state on these terms, but one that supports a basic universal income.

This kind of theory can accommodate a robust public health state in the following way. Some projected health state is required for our future goals (condition 1). In the immediate term, individuals' future goals require they be healthy today in order to prepare, gather resources, and engage in community (including participating in politics) to be able to achieve their goals. They will need, moreover, to be able to maintain their health through to their goals, and potentially beyond. Achieving our goals, including nonhealth goals, will often require a particular health state (condition 2). Importantly, these are an individual's health goals, and are arguably necessary for them to advance their interests, independent of whether their health advances the goals of others (condition 3). We all have a deep personal connection to our own health states, whatever those are.

Unlike some liberal theories that ask us to envision a world where we don't know our health states going forward, Moehler's theory does not require us to adopt an uncertain (e.g., probability blind or equiprobable) view of health.[45] It does not require, for example, that we imagine the possibility that we could be born into a body that has a congenital disorder. Rather, Moehler's theory assumes only that individuals know who they are in real life, and the social and economic circumstances of their society.

They are further assumed to be uncertain only about the particular cases of conflict in which they might become involved, the future, and their precise positions in each of these situations.[46]

This kind of public health state can be quite robust. Let's return to the principal focus of health security: communicable disease. There are a broad range of communicable diseases to which individuals are vulnerable, even in relatively developed societies: recall the US experiences up to 50,000 deaths from flu per year,[47] or up to one Vietnam War of influenza deaths every year. These infectious diseases can and do frustrate the goals of individuals in a range of ways, from death to time spent not pursuing other activities while recovering.

However, a coordination problem arises, regardless of the moral commitments of the agents in question, in which routine interactions for business or pleasure form a possible route of transmission of those diseases, and which without an agent's interests would be frustrated. That is, absent the public health state, our conditions can look a lot like the state of nature in some very important respects. Few rational agents want to become sick with an infectious disease, and while in many areas they might be willing to risk it absent other options, there are compelling reasons to accept a state that handles the control of communicable diseases so that individual agents can better achieve their goals, and achieve them with less risk. While communicable diseases are the primary focus of this book, there are other areas where risk sharing is in the interests of a very broad coalition of parties, including environmental and occupational health risks.

This, moreover, provides a very robust emphasis on the nation-state's health infrastructure in aid of public health. COVID-19 gives us a great example of how robust this kind of arrangement might be once fully described. In an op-ed in June 2020, Luciana Borio, vice president at In-Q-Tel—the venture capital arm of the Central Intelligence Agency, and thus securitized health if ever there was—noted that clinical trials to generate knowledge about COVID-19 and develop treatments and novel therapeutics were hampered by fragmented healthcare systems.[48] Borio, while lauding the Randomized Evaluation of COVID-19 Therapy (RECOVERY) trial platform that provided rapid and robust data on therapies for COVID-19, did not explore its mobilization of the UK National Health Service, and that the existence of the NHS in terms of common standards of care provision and a unified health records system made such innovative trials possible.[49] A comprehensive and unified healthcare system is itself an asset to the coordination problem of health security. Independent of our other moral commitments, from a self-interested, instrumentally rational perspective, universal healthcare *is* pandemic preparedness. In addition to solving issues around risk pooling that can arise with more fragmented health systems, it solves key coordination issues that may arise when the first notification of a public health crisis comes from a patient reporting symptoms, to responding quickly to novel diseases through high-quality data generation.

A common concern in these kinds of arguments is what we do about free riders. That is, the degree to which these kinds of state measures are vulnerable to exploitation by individuals who do not pay into the system, but instead simply draw from it. But here, a robust public health system can be justified on what Moehler calls "productivist grounds," referring to the broad welfare states of social democratic states such as those in the Nordic League.[50] This is because the preventative effects of a robust public health system are extremely net cost saving. They benefit producers, including employers, in virtue of reducing the burden of disease on the population that causes losses in productivity. Seasonal influenza, for example, exerts an economic burden of approximately $11.2 billion on the USA, of which approximately 70 percent is due to indirect costs such as productivity loss from 20 million or so sick people a year.[51] Even if there are free riders, the sheer volume of lost productivity from even vaccine-preventable infectious diseases can justify substantial investment in public health.

Likewise, public health can protect social fabric writ large, with considerable gains in productive labor that overwhelm free-riding concerns. This enters into condition 4, and the satisfaction of interests in a way that secures long-term peaceful cooperation. Pandemics can debilitate states, depleting economies and undermining the capacity for individuals to fulfill their basic needs. The structure of communities can be undermined through long term public health effects resulting from disease pandemics, including lack of access to education, other medical care, and basic services. In this way, the public health state is justified just in case it provides a *security* against catastrophic events that undermine the possibility of long-term peaceful cooperation.

Finally, robust public health in principle provides a mechanism for accounting for the considerable unpaid labor that goes into supporting fragmented or undervalued public health systems. Taking care of sick children or adult relatives, time off work to attend doctor's visits or to recover, individuals bearing costs of measures to prevent the transmission of disease—all of these constitute a form of unpaid labor that prevents individuals from otherwise pursuing their own ends. This, on the one hand, relates to the kinds of social arrangement a broad set of individuals can agree to above—there are broad segments of society who enter into these unpaid labor arrangements, including everyone who raises children. But this also folds into productivist reasons to enhance the public health state to allow individuals to enter into these otherwise unpaid circumstances to prevent the spread of disease: rather than worrying about free riders, the amount of uncompensated labor that goes into responding to the routine spread of infectious disease is immense relative to the costs, I suspect, of supporting individuals to prevent its spread.

Two final points are relevant here. The first pertains to negotiation. Given that Moehler's account doesn't assume an ideal negotiating position, should we expect to a public health state to be agreed to in the kind of world we have? I'll set aside politically enforced barriers to participation until the final chapter, but for now it is worth showing why a coalition of citizens can be constructed to support this strategy. That is, the fabric of our society can help describe precisely why actual rational agents would endorse this vision of the public health state. For 26 percent of Americans, it is a disability. This includes the almost 14 percent of Americans who have a mobility disorder, and all members of the community who engage in unpaid labor to support them.[52] For almost 60 percent of Americans, it is a chronic disease such as heart disease, cancer, lung disease, or diabetes. It is the 43.5 million people in the US who will have children between the ages of 15 and 50, and their partners. Most all of these individuals have an interest not simply in medical care, but in public health measures that prevent illness and provide a mechanism to prevent its spread in a mostly voluntaristic way. I assume that in most other nations, the numbers above may change, and additional groups may be folded into this account, but the general sketch of a coalition remains the same. The number of people with an interest in a robust public health state simply overwhelms the people who have little to no interest in it.

Note I am not suggesting healthism—preoccupation with personal health as a primary, and often *the* primary, focus for the definition and achievement of well-being[53]—is the rational or moral option here. Lots of things are required for a good life, and no good life need be the same on my account.

But many of the things individuals value about their lives can impose risk on themselves. This might include certain kinds of food, drink, drug use, travel, hobbies, or athletic, sexual, social, and other activities that people engage in that carry some kind of health risk. But here, the need for robust public health infrastructure is at its most stark, and the negotiating aspect features heavily. With rare exception, no one group of individuals that has an interest in being protected by the state from one public health risk, or supported if they incur the negative outcomes resulting from the pursuit of another, has the power to otherwise demand of others that they refrain from a risky practice or pursuit. Individuals who prefer food that carries a higher risk of foodborne illnesses likely lack the power to demand that people who like to hike outdoors, where they might encounter parasites, are not covered by the public health state. But both have an interest in public health mechanisms that permit those activities but invest in detecting and responding to them as needed. Thus, surveillance of foodborne outbreaks and of seasonal parasite densities are both part of the contract, whereas banning oysters and raw sprouts are not. In fact, there is an advantage to both groups to negotiate for the protection of their activities, say, modern capital, whose leaders may prefer not to incur the taxes to pay for more robust public health. Just as with disability, or childrearing, all rational agents who have an interest in securing long-term cooperation have strong interests in forming these kinds of health coalitions.

A final set of individuals who enter into this coalition are individuals who are at risk for losing employment through the spread of disease. First, in April 2020, roughly 14 percent of US workers were unemployed, half of whom never returned to the workforce. Second, individuals experienced long-term harm from disease even if they survived: an international survey of "long COVID" sequelae found that of respondents with COVID-19, 45 percent required reduced work time compared to pre-illness, and another 22 percent left the workforce.[54] Finally, individuals experienced the year-to-year insecurity that arises from a lack of access to paid sick leave, or sick-leave policies that do not provide substantial, feasible access to time off for major illness. These individuals will recognize that living in a society that broadly protects individuals from becoming sick is in their interests. I suspect they will also have personal experience with the idea that access to paid sick leave is itself a form of infectious disease control, and immediately grasp why countries with paid time off are estimated to have up to 40 percent lower influenza burdens.[55] But between these groups, individuals suffering from chronic illness, individuals with disabilities, and individuals with care obligations, we can imagine a coalition that promotes an incredibly robust public health state—and has the relative bargaining power to enforce it.

This account of public health assumes nothing about the substantive moral commitments of individuals. It is unlikely to fully satisfy the moral demands of libertarians, contract theorists, or utilitarians. However, it provides a structure that all should be able to agree to as part of an effort to maintain long-term peaceful cooperation, and insofar as they hold beliefs that preclude them dissolving the social contract altogether. It will also satisfy the interests of individuals who, in all likelihood, do not maintain a single coherent normative theory of the state, but also possess those qualities described above.

This view of the public health state has two levels. The first level strongly promotes a rights or interests-promoting account of public health. This is because while individuals have a fundamental interest in maintaining their health (in some state) in advancing their goals, they will not agree to a social contract that does not protect their existence as separate agents and does not allow them to satisfy their basic needs. Those needs, moreover, may be divergent. Because the precise, substantive value of health may differ for individuals, public health must be able to account for individuals for whom health is intrinsically valuable or is its own benefit. But it must also account for (I suspect, but cannot be certain, is much a larger set of) individuals for whom health is a means to an end, and where those ends diverge radically: from elite sportspeople who require an extremely high level of performance beyond the subsistence needs of their bodies, to people with disabilities for whom guarding against certain pathologies and maintaining access to their central projects and autonomy is centrally important. It must also deal with individuals for whom health is minimally important, and important merely to facilitate their lives and non-health goals. The people who "don't care about their health" are, paradoxically, likely to be the healthiest among us (likely from brute luck) in that they don't notice their own good health.

The second level of public health, on the other hand, looks highly securitized on its face. This level of public health seeks to protect against severe health events that may damage society, temporarily or permanently, to the degree that individuals have a preference that those events be prevented or mitigated, and against which individuals are uncertain about their place and outcomes in future such events. This level of public health is securitized in the sense that it seeks, like the institution of national security, to maintain the structure of the state against exogenous threats.

This provides a strong reason basis for health security as, effectively, the militant arm of public health. Note, however, that this does not establish a theory of the state that sees health security as part of *the national security state* against human aggressors. Rather, it establishes the state as a legitimate authority from which to provide public health in securing the aims of individuals against external threats. What form that takes is a further issue to resolve.

Objections

Two objections arise here, which are important to map out now but whose resolution I will leave for later in the book. The first is what we do if we loosen some of the conditions of Moehler's account further, and in particular the fourth condition about long-term cooperation. Surely, someone could say while pointing to the mess that is COVID-19, there are plenty of individuals who at this stage would rather break long-term cooperation than maintain it. In these cases, their relative bargaining positions would be less important because they are not interested in bargaining, or because they are powerful enough that they control an outsized share of power. Examples readers might suppose here are anti-mask protests,[56] or violent white nationalist groups threatening to intentionally infect their victims, or the QAnon movement and other conspiracy theorists that prefer to disrupt society despite its impact on public health.

Moehler has a partial answer to this, and he acknowledges the possibility of this in general terms:

> In cases of conflict . . . the parties to a conflict are so severely negatively affected by the points of contention that, if the conflicts remain unresolved, they are prepared to engage in destructive actions and threaten peaceful long-term cooperation, because they consider such actions to be more beneficial to them than remaining in their current situation. To be clear, typically there is a continuum from peaceful cooperation to the mere rejection of cooperation to socially disruptive but nonviolent resolution to explicitly violent conflict resolution.[57]

Moehler's solution, then, is that in most cases rational individuals will prefer peace to conflict because the costs of conflict are very high. In some cases, individuals might not be rational, but in others they may prefer conflict because the state of affairs of their negotiations is so poor that conflict becomes *preferred* to peaceful resolution.

I buy this account, though what we ought to do about it is a more complex matter. Part of this, however, returns us to coalition building. Given the broad set of individuals who have an interest in a robust public health state, it seems that a key challenge for that coalition is exerting pressure on individuals who do not have the same interest. While this pressure might involve persuasion, it might—to return us to the struggles of disability and HIV/AIDS activists—also involve confrontation. This is consistent with Moehler's account, though I suspect it will not be a happy conclusion for some.

This dovetails into the major concern about negotiation, and falls into what political philosophers would call "nonideal theory." The issue at stake is that currently, political and social incentives are arranged in such a way that the coalitions mentioned are largely fragmented. How do we get not just to a point of collective action to agree to something like the above, in all its inevitable complexity, but do so in the existing political system?

I have some suggestions to this, which I lay out in the final chapter. I take the nonideal question to be broader than this book, despite being a through line in some of the ethical and political philosophical claims I make throughout. What is clear, however, is that considerable support exists for broad public health promotion, including institutional changes outside of public health proper that would support the public health state. Universal healthcare, free or subsidized education, paid time off, and living wages are all connected to the public's health, and if I understand my colleagues in political science, all receive broad support from citizens despite their nature as political hot buttons. The overarching question is one of how we build coalitions in that environment.

A second objection would be to contest how rights respecting this system would be. This dovetails partly with the securitization angle, in terms of the capacity for communities to buy in to the most egregious government programs as they did during the war on terror. But it also dovetails with the history of public health, and the public's willingness to accept draconian public health measures so long as they target people other than themselves.

A preliminary response to this is that, as ideal theory, I accept that in practice actual negotiations may take a different tack. But I note that the architecture of this theory provides a robust degree of safety that satisfies concerns individuals have about public health measures—there are ways to satisfy the aims of more restrictive public health measures, if we have the imagination and will to act. This leaves open room for more liberty-centric public health practices that are seen not only as the best means to solve public health and view securitized practice as a last resort but to promote the self-interest of other parties as well. This does not mean that individuals, presented with evidence, may not decide to impose their will on others regardless. But as mentioned above, the response to this may be to make that imposition untenable as a means to resolve conflict.

Conclusion

In this chapter, I establish a general legitimacy of the public health state: the role of the structure of basic institutions of the state in maintaining the public's health. I outlined a broad contractarian argument for why diverse and deeply pluralistic societies can consent to an arrangement of institutions aimed at this goal, with an appeal first to the role health plays in individual lives, and then through an appeal to the role public health plays in maintaining the possibility of peaceful, long-term cooperation in a society.

The next step required is to justify public health as uniquely deserving of an explicit institutional role in modern states. This argument will turn on the nature of the threat in public health, with a focus on the latter level of the public health state: protection against threats that threaten long-term stability. Through that, I will show how we can account for other public health operations, albeit at different levels of decision making. But in particular, the role of the largest coherent collective actor—currently the nation-state—as the authority comes into its own in cases where stability is threatened.

6 Justly Declaring an Emergency

The COVID-19 epidemic arrived on December 30, 2019, when China notified WHO of a cluster of pneumonia cases. It would take another month for the outbreak, however, to become officially an emergency in the eyes of the international community, when the WHO director general declared COVID-19 a public health emergency of international concern. In the lead up to this decision, as in previous outbreaks, considerable attention was paid to when, and why, the emergency committee at WHO would issue its recommendation of a public health emergency of international concern to the director general, and what the result would be.

The declaration of the public health emergency of international concern was fraught for a couple of reasons. On the one hand, it was clear to observers that COVID-19, which had spread to more than a dozen other countries at that point, had long posed a risk to the international community.[1] On the other, the severe lockdown in Hubei province a week earlier raised fears that countries would react in regressive ways, potentially even those detrimental to a pandemic response.[2] The lack of rationale provided to WHO by China for instituting public health measures beyond WHO recommendations, something required under IHR, raised fears that international norms would fall by the wayside in the panic.[3] On both counts, the why and when of the declaration mattered not just for definitional purposes, but as authorization for what was and was not an acceptable response to a crisis.

This chapter deals with the ethics of declaring a public health emergency. The previous chapters described the impersonal account of disease as entailing a last resort before implementing emergency measures that violate the rights of citizens, and the fundamental tension at the heart of health security arising from the structure of the state as a legitimate authority in promoting public health. These provide a strong presumption against infringing on rights in the pursuit of public health goals. Powers exercised during public health crises can be severe, tend to disproportionately harm the most vulnerable members of society, and can harm communities for generations. They are, moreover, frequently exercised through the executive powers of government, and can be difficult to hold accountable or resist when used inappropriately.

In this chapter, I consolidate the principles discussed in previous chapters into an account of a just declaration of a public health emergency. I begin first with a note on the definitional ambiguities surrounding what constitutes a public health emergency. I then clarify the work of the previous chapters establishing legitimate authority and last resort criteria as the criteria for declaring a just public health emergency.

I then turn to the remaining criteria. I distinguish between proportionality and necessity as important and distinct concerns in declaring a public health emergency, and their interaction with last resort criteria. I finish with a comment on how the chance of success, and the possibility that a health emergency might make certain threats worse, could provide reasons not to declare a public health emergency. I then consider objections, and importantly the possibility of using liberty-limiting public health measures outside of an emergency.

A Problem of Definitions

Little literature exists on what exactly constitutes a public health emergency. This is a significant omission in public health ethics, and more so because of the proliferation of competing and varied accounts of a public health emergency in law, as described in chapter 3. This significance lies in questions of the ethical implications of declaring an emergency, and in particular what powers it authorizes the use of in aid of resolving an emergency.

WHO is a good place to start. A PHEIC is defined as "an extraordinary event which is determined to constitute a public health risk to other States through the international spread of disease and to potentially require a coordinated international response," formulated when a situation arises that is "serious, sudden, unusual or unexpected," which "carries implications for public health beyond the affected state's national border" and "may require immediate international action."[4] Within that, important elements emerge: the risk of transnational spread; the requirement for a coordinated international response; and a serious, sudden, or unexpected event.[5]

The PHEIC, however, is neither the arbiter nor model of the public health emergency. In the United States, for example, a number of definitions exist and may differ depending on the scope and level of government actor. The Stafford Act defines a "major disaster" as "natural catastrophe (including any hurricane, tornado, storm, high water, wind-driven water, tidal wave, tsunami, earthquake, volcanic eruption, landslide, mudslide, snowstorm, or drought)."[6] But the act defines an defines emergency as "any occasion or instance for which, in the determination of the President, Federal assistance is needed to supplement State and local efforts and capabilities to save lives and to protect property and public health and safety, or to lessen or avert the threat of a catastrophe in any part of the United States. The Public Health Service Act states that the secretary of the Department of Health and Human Services is authorized to declare a public health emergency on finding that "1) a disease or disorder presents a public emergency, or 2) a public health emergency, including significant outbreaks of infectious diseases or bioterrorist attacks, otherwise exists."[7] However, the same act does not actually define what constitutes that emergency.

The Model Act designed by Gostin and colleagues provides an outline for a health emergency as an occurrence or imminent threat of an illness or health condition that:

1. is believed to be caused by any of the following:

   i. bioterrorism;
   ii. the appearance of a novel or previously controlled or eradicated infectious agent or biological toxin;
   iii. [a natural disaster;]
   iv. [a chemical attack or accidental release; or]
   v. [a nuclear attack or accident]; and

2. poses a high probability of any of the following harms:

   i. a large number of deaths in the affected population;
   ii. a large number of serious or long-term disabilities in the affected population; or
   iii. widespread exposure to an infectious or toxic agent that poses a significant risk of substantial future harm to a large number of people in affected population.[8]

As I explained in chapter 3, however, the definition in the Model Act rarely finds its way into state acts in whole or in part. Some states retain the wording of the Model Act, such as Indiana, which defines it as "occurrence or imminent threat of widespread or severe injury, or loss of life or property resulting from any natural phenomenon or human act, including an epidemic and public health emergency."[9] Others, such as Massachusetts and Florida, have no definition of what counts as an emergency.

Rather than merely assess which jurisdictions do or do not define emergencies, however, we can assess what kind of properties best describe a public health emergency. First, the structure of nation-states is strongly determinant of an emergency declaration. Not only do individual nations differ from the WHO in what counts as an emergency, but individual substate jurisdictions within those nations differ, including between each other, about what constitutes a health emergency. This reaffirms the ameliorative, critical piece of this project: to engage with health security with an eye toward institutional reform.

Second, while commonalities exist between definitions of a public health emergency, such as the seriousness of the event, even those commonalities are vague. What constitutes a serious event, or one requiring mobilization, or significant risk, is far from clear. This is not necessarily avoidable but motivates further analysis. Moreover, different legal histories among jurisdictions may mean that features of these terms may be interpreted in divergent ways. So even if we have the same definition, the effects may be different.

The presence of language around a public health emergency does not just describe what such an emergency constitutes as a descriptive feature of the world. Declaring a public health emergency is an action that, once performed, creates certain kinds of outcomes for the world. The relationship between the definition, the declaration, and its outcomes is an important social-scientific phenomenon, but what that relationship ought to be is also an important philosophical question.

What Is a Public Health Emergency (And What Should It Be)?

Rather than a formal definition, I present a conceptual framework that distinguishes between what properties public health emergencies might have, and the reasons we declare emergencies. I do so quickly, to consolidate previous discussions in earlier chapters.

To the first, a descriptive account of an emergency can be read from my account of disease as a security issue. Public health emergencies are first exigent and immediate. They come on quickly, and before a conventional political response is capable of addressing them. This property is contingent on how good our political responses are, but we can imagine that even the best designed political systems are vulnerable to shocks they cannot absorb.

The second is the harm that arises. Public health emergencies can kill or otherwise harm large numbers of people. These numbers can be so large that, like in war, they can appear to be indiscriminate. Public health will never absolutely be able to prevent disease and death, but the magnitude of the excess harm that constitutes an emergency is a threat to the continuation of the social fabric, in addition to the health of individuals. Countries or communities might survive these events—they need not be existential threats—but are left changed by them, potentially for generations.

Third, and related to the above, is the capacity for response. Even relatively small infectious disease outbreaks can overwhelm a weak or underprepared health system. The Ebola virus disease outbreak in Liberia was so challenging in part because Liberia, recovering from a civil war in 2003, had approximately 298 physicians for its 4.5 million population,[10] and lost 8 percent of its healthcare workforce over the course of the pandemic.[11] While this is not the only measure of vulnerability that is relevant, it is indicative of the kind of damage that a disease can do when it strikes a weak health system. Exigency, harm, and capacity are related properties that capture central features of what makes public health issues into public health emergencies.

This, however, is not what constitutes *declaring* a public health emergency. Rather, the above recapitulates the threat that may prompt the declaration of an emergency. But not all emerging threats justify declaring a public health emergency. Like a war, a declaration of emergency is not a natural phenomenon, but a choice by an institution or state. It is moreover a choice that implicates states (singular or plural), a disease event, and the people caught in the middle.

What a declaration of an emergency typically does is change the power structure of a state. This happens in three ways. First, it relaxes executive powers to perform public health measures during an emergency, and the enforcement powers of states to ensure compliance with those orders. This may include removing or withholding licensing to perform certain activities, the use of criminal justice powers and law enforcement, and even the deployment of military units to perform operations in aid of an emergency. This is a wide variety of enforcement options, but part of this breadth is arguably intentional because it provides an executive with discretion to use the means they deem necessary to accomplish their goals.

These powers typically enable the infringement of civil, political, social, and economic rights or liberties otherwise protected by law, in order to respond to a threat. This typically lasts for the duration of the emergency, is authorized for a particular set of representatives of the executive or legislative bodies of a state and is overseen by judiciaries for appeals and contests of certain powers. The paradigm of the kind of powers in use is quarantine, in which a person's freedom of movement is curtailed because they are suspected of being exposed to an infectious disease.[12] While quarantine of humans might be used in nonemergent scenarios as well, it is typically found in emergencies as a loosening of traditional powers of healthcare institutions and government. Where quarantine differs from isolation in healthcare facilities is that isolation is the confinement of someone who is already sick and thus clearly poses a danger to themselves and others; where it differs from prison is that people under quarantine are not charged or guilty of a crime.[13] Emergency powers provide a mechanism for this otherwise impermissible or at least highly restricted use of state power in a public health emergency, though hopefully not one that is unlimited.

Second, a declaration of emergency allows the mobilization of resources to respond to a threat. Resource requests may be freed from budget constraints brought about by typical governance processes. Existing resources may be reallocated from other projects by the executive or its representative, such as a public health commissioner or chief medical officer. And an emergency may authorize the deployment or requisition of specific emergency supplies that are set aside for such an event.

Finally, public health emergencies may trigger changes in the regulatory powers used by the state to govern the practice of medicine or other essential fields, to allow them to operate in ways they might not otherwise in aid of an emergency response. A public health emergency may justify, for example, loosening existing regulatory requirements that are otherwise in place to ensure public safety, such as allowing emergency authorizations of therapeutics or vaccines. We might also see looser privacy regulations to increase the speed and breadth of health information sharing in order to mobilize contact tracing and other interventions.

Just Cause

What an emergency is, and does, connects us to the moral basis of a public health emergency. An appropriately designed public health state is robust, and has strong, rights-preserving obligations to prevent public health emergencies from arising. What an emergency declaration allows is for the state to disrupt that order temporarily to protect the community. That kind of disruption, however, has to be for the right reason. In war, this reason is the just cause.

Previously, I provided a list that tracked the correspondence between the orthodox view of public health ethics and just war theory. Below, table 6.1 has been updated to reflect the work of the previous three chapters in establishing a last resort and legitimate authority as important features of a securitized public health ethics. I established the impersonal account of threat and connected it to the principle of last resort. The communicable disease threat posed by individual humans does not motivate strong defensive permissions, and thus should play little role in the acts of the public health state in responding to communicable diseases. We can thus, I argued, consider the public as similar to noncombatants under the war analogy. Their rights against interference are not waived in virtue of the risk they pose to others, and this provides a strong claim against others to refrain from using coercive or other harmful means to prosecute a response to a public health crisis. Critically, because of the magnitude of the harms and deprivations

Table 6.1
Correspondence between just war theory and public health ethics (update 1)

Temporal/contextual feature	Just war theory	Public health ethics
Declaring an emergency	Just cause	??
	Last resort	Last resort
	Legitimate authority	Legitimate authority
	Right intention	??
	Reasonable success	??
	Proportionality	??
During the emergency	Necessity	Effectiveness/necessity
	Proportionality	Proportionality
	Discrimination	Least infringement
	??	Public justification

public health emergencies can inflict on the public, the state has an obligation to ensure that the conditions that led to public health emergencies are addressed, such that a public health emergency response arose as a last resort.

I then identified the basis of the state as the ultimate provider for the public's health, based on a thin account of moral consensus in which self-interested actors could plausibly bargain with a state that supported a robust public health apparatus not just for protection against health emergencies, but the protection of a robust range of public health functions. This state, I claimed, supported the social institution of public health as part of its moral function, and thus possessed the authority to enact public health policy as part of traditional democratic means, and to declare and react to public health crises.

These two principles in military ethics join additional criteria, including just cause and right intention. I think, however, that the latter of these is unnecessary for an account of just health security. Right intention, historically, has been focused on the dispositions of the people going to war: Christians in particular, in early versions of the theory, were expected to refrain from sentiments like lust for revenge and to treat the vanquished with mercy.[14] While it is absolutely possible, as in the case of vilifying minority populations, to act in public health with bad intentions, it seems unlikely that our dispositions matter if we accept the impersonal account of disease. It might reflect something poor about our dispositions for us to hate viruses or fungi, but it does not seem to track the declaration of a public health emergency in the same way as if our enemy were persons. And if we have identified persons as our threat, we have likely erred not simply in right intention, but in the last resort, legitimate authority and just cause.

This, then, brings us to the just cause for a public health emergency. A just cause arises in which

> *Just cause*: the just cause for a public health emergency is to respond to a threat to the public's health that threatens mass harm or community stability, is exigent, and is overwhelming.

Not all health crises are necessarily public health emergencies, and some might be prosecuted for the wrong reasons. Take the Ebola virus disease outbreak of 2014. In Connecticut, Governor Malloy issued a "cautionary" public health emergency declaration on October 16, 2014, which remained in place until April 1, 2016.[15] During that time, individuals were quarantined independent of their exposure to EVD, including individuals returning from the African continent who had never been near an affected region.[16] While right intention would be difficult to determine for a governor's office, on its face the declaration was made in a state that had never experienced a case of Ebola, had a healthcare system more than capable of responding to a single or even a handful of cases, and a functioning public health department for a disease that was only transmissible when a patient was showing symptoms. Given the CDC's orders at the time—which recommended only screening and ongoing temperature checks for individuals returning from areas with known cases of Ebola virus disease—there was no reason to declare a public health emergency. There was simply no threat, relevantly defined, to the area in question. Ebola virus disease may have been, in an immediate sense, a public health emergency satisfying just cause in Western Africa—but not in Connecticut, or Australia, or the United Kingdom, where the threat did not exist.

Note, however, that a different kind of declaration might have been permissible. Sometimes scholars of war refer to "defense of another" as just cause. Here, the declaration of war by a state is not to protect itself, but to protect an ally. It may be permissible, as long as other criteria of just health security are satisfied, to declare a public health emergency in aid of assisting another in responding to an exigent, harmful, overwhelming threat. But note that if this was the kind of declaration the state of Connecticut, or another nation, had made, activities like the one above would need to be justified on defending another nation from the threat—and here the actions taken would have to reflect that cause.

Consider, alternately, the ongoing overdose epidemic in the United States. The states of Massachusetts, Florida, Alaska, Arizona, Virginia, and Maryland, by 2017, had declared public health emergencies in response to this epidemic.[17] In the first case, the declaration of a public health emergency in Massachusetts by Governor Baker served to restrict access to opioid analgesics and redirect funding from other projects to the overdose crisis. Massachusetts attempted to overrule the FDA's approval of a hydrocodone-only pill, which was later struck down for exceeding the state's authority. It also provided some funding for the emergency purchase of naloxone by the state, and for civil commitment of individuals with opioid use disorder.[18]

The overdose epidemic, however, is difficult to justify as a public health emergency on the basis of just cause. It is certainly harmful and might arguably be considered overwhelming. But it is not exigent in the sense that a justified threat entails, because it is *not one threat*. Housing crises, job crises, mental health crises—all of these are ongoing and have been for decades, not only in the state of Massachusetts but around the United States. The crisis that is the referent of these public health emergency declarations, moreover, is the deaths from overdose associated with opioids. But these "deaths of despair" are not necessarily solvable within the strictures of the—by design—temporary provisions of a public health emergency. A public health emergency that never ends because it is a symptom of a larger political system is not a public health emergency, relevantly defined. The source of the emergency is endogenous and political, not exogenous and emergent. It is almost a public health civil conflict, declared by government against its own failures.

This is not to say we should do nothing about the overdose crisis: just that it is not the right kind of public health issue against which to deploy emergency powers. The use of emergency powers here reflects a lack of political will and due care for fellow citizens. Writing this in Lowell, Massachusetts, less than ten miles from the epicenter of the overdose epidemic in the state, the problems of the Merrimack Valley and surrounds are almost a century old, from the collapse of meaningful work to the lack of attention paid to the northern part of the state for redevelopment and investment, to the fragmented governance of the state. But this is not the kind of crisis for which emergency powers, and the disruption they can cause, are justified.

In some cases, however, there may be structural or local factors that are the appropriate triggers for just cause. This is the health security equivalent of a preemptive war. We could imagine a large, emergent cluster of avian flu infecting a poultry flock that, while normally well cared for in correspondence with appropriate surveillance and animal care, leads to the transmission of the disease through the family that runs the farm. Rapid contact tracing by public health officials identifies the existence of two cases in contacts of the family, but who do not report dealing with poultry in close contact. A trigger here is a novel, highly pathogenic flu strain showing signs of secondary human transmission where it normally only affects individuals in direct contact with animal reservoirs. We might think that preempting this possible pandemic (given what we know about the potential for pandemic strains of flu to spread) is a sufficient, reasonable aim to motivate an emergency, but it is a borderline case and would need to be balanced against other criteria.

Prevention, on the other hand, arises in war when one attacks a potential enemy in order to undermine their ability to one day attack you in the future. It is widely understood to violate the just cause criterion in war, but that case is more difficult to understand in the context of public health ethics. After all, preventing the causative agent of a communicable disease from causing a disease outbreak appears to be precisely the kind of goal public health should have. But framed in the context of declaring a public health emergency, wariness about prevention makes more sense. This is because prevention in routine public health is considerably different in terms of the kinds of institutional power wielded by the state under a health emergency declaration. It is less about whether prevention is a good or bad thing, and more about whether prevention can ever be a reason to authorize the powers of a public health emergency.

Here, I think there is a robust case to be made against most kinds of prevention using the tools of a public health emergency. This lies at the intersection of just cause and the principle of last resort. If a public health emergency declaration is used on a potential public health issue that has not yet risen to or is imminently approaching the level of threat that would otherwise provide a just cause, then the principle of last resort is very unlikely to have been fulfilled as well. Moreover, even in some rare situation where there may really be no other options available to a state in dealing with a public health issue, it might still not satisfy just cause because the institutional arrangements of the robust public health state will sometimes support the autonomy of non-dominated individuals to engage in activities that might increase that public health risk. I have few ideas as to what kind of situation this latter case might entail, but we shouldn't rule out under our contractarian scheme that some potential future public health emergencies, even with a motivated, informed, rationally self-interested population, will be tolerated by that population. A key component of the rights theory that undergirds this contractarian scheme is that while other values can at times override civil, social, political, and economic rights, those rights are at least somewhat insensitive to consequences. The mere possibility that a certain set of acts could lead to a public health threat large enough to motivate a public health emergency is not in itself a reason to declare a public health emergency as a means of prevention.

Proportionality

Proportionality is a critical condition of declaring a public health emergency, and like the declaration of war is part of paired, parallel conditions.

In *ad bellum* considerations in war, this pair takes the form of proportionality and last resort; in *in bello*, proportionality and necessity.[19]

These conditions are paralleled in an account of just health security that takes seriously the role of the public health state. Proportionality and last resort are partly independent. One could imagine a public health emergency where the benefits of intervening through an emergency declaration outweigh the costs, but where the presence of other options violates the last resort condition. Alternatively, an emergency of last resort may conceivably be one in which the benefits of action are disproportionately outweighed by the costs.

At the same time, the last resort condition is related to the proportionality criterion through our decision process. This is because to assess last resort, we need to have a sense of our options and their relative costs and benefits. Not all those potential trade-offs will be permissible under a principle of last resort, but we have to know our options to establish it.

A perennial problem for public health ethics is that the benefits and harms of a public health action are not always indexable against each other, or indexable at all. There is an obvious sense in which we can weigh potential lives lost, or saved, against each other; or life years, adjusted for quality or disability. But these measures may not be able to be compared against rights in a way that is easily computable, such as X deaths are sufficient to justify Y rights infringements.[20] Likewise, the economic impacts of pandemics and responses are important, and some economic calculations may be especially important in terms of diseases that do not kill but may temporarily or even permanently impair those infected at the cost of productivity in a state—which can, in turn, affect everything from employment to food productivity to health service provision. But it is unlikely that indexing lives against dollars is advisable as the only strategy in thinking about the balance of benefits and harms in declaring a public health emergency.

Likewise, the mainstay proxies for value in public health, such as excess deaths, may be outweighed by other considerations such as the values of community integrity and autonomy. Consider a disease epidemic that threatens indigenous communities. While the morbidity and mortality of tribal members is obviously important, we should be wary if this is only thing that matters to the state. Long-standing norms around tribal sovereignty and a commitment to solving a public health issue, even a very serious one, using the values integral to the community might outweigh even an increase in lives saved through an emergency regime. This is the case even though in practice I suspect respecting indigenous sovereignty is likely to be the most effective as a public health measure. While tribal nations worldwide have suffered grievously from COVID-19, they have also produced responses to the pandemic that have matched and at times exceeded state and federal responses, and lent credence to claims that their comparatively high death tolls are in the main due to the long-standing injustices they have endured and in which they began the pandemic, and not the quality of their immediate response.[21]

Just war theory includes a separate criterion for a reasonable chance for success. In the context of public health, however, I think this criterion would be better served as a procedural component of proportionality. Assessing the risks and benefits requires not only their magnitude and kind, but the likelihood of certain kinds of benefits/harms coming to pass if we choose to make or refrain from making an emergency declaration. In war, there is a possibility that an invading enemy might be so powerful that resisting them, so long as they are not waging a war of extermination, might be so futile that it may be better to lose one's sovereignty—even if only temporarily—than endure the catastrophe of a war.

But the kinds of crises to which health security responds do not work in quite the same way. It is hard to imagine the following: a disease exigent and harmful to the extent it presents a just cause, a proportionate response, and a last resort; but one for which we have no chance of resisting and should rely solely on the means of conventional public health to respond. I take it that should this occur, it is *because* responding to the disease will be outlandishly harmful to the public. But either that is justified under the proportionality requirement (some kind of "zombie apocalypse" or other existential threat) or it isn't (because it isn't that serious). Viruses don't accept surrender, so the idea that there is a conditional threat in which there is a proportionate capitulation is not on the table like it is in war.

Force Short of (Public Health) War

One obvious objection to the structure provided here is why we *shouldn't* be radically preemptive. After all, in public health of all fields an ounce of prevention beats a pound of cure. Why not defeat the microbial enemy before it even has a chance to reveal itself?

The simple answer to this is grounded in a thoroughgoing appreciation of the doctrine of last resort, and to recanvas the impacts of public health emergencies on the citizenry. Public health emergencies can be devastating, ripping apart families and destroying communities as nonpharmaceutical interventions are deployed to break the transmission of disease; depressing economies for years; placing others at risk through high-stakes healthcare; and destroying the mental and physical health of first responders. It is true that we should do as much as we can to prevent an emergency from arising but utilizing the logic of emergencies to prevent other emergencies is dangerous in its own right. It erodes trust in authorities, and its measures can backfire in the process.

Here too, just war theory can provide guidance. In recent years, just war theory has developed, in response to low-level armed engagements, a theory of *jus ad vim*, or "force short of war." The theory emerged with the fourth edition of Walzer's *Just and Unjust Wars* which, in 2006, attempted to address the war in and occupation of Iraq. Walzer's addition to his canonical account of theory is intended to think through the role of decisive, lethal force in preventing war, though it has in virtue of its applied subject matter caused considerable controversy.[22]

Much of *jus ad vim* is developed along the same lines as *jus in bello*, which as we have seen is broadly homologous with the orthodox view of public health ethics. A critical difference is that *jus ad vim* includes a criterion of last resort, and a unique criterion: probability of de-escalation.[23] Using force short of war, like a drone strike, is a risky affair. The history of the drone war is one in which entire regions of the world have been destabilized and thrown into further conflict as a result of the use of force by America and its allies.[24] While Peter Daszak may have been right in that we do send out the drones in response to terrorism, he is much too cavalier on the wisdom of doing so. We often make things much worse. This is why de-escalation is so important: the purpose of *jus ad vim* is to prevent the horrors of war, not drive nations toward them.

This is the crucial issue in prevention through executive or unrestrained government power in public health. For a public health emergency response to occur outside a formal declaration of emergency, there would have to be a reasonable expectation that our actions would lead us to avoid having to declare a public health emergency in the future. But, because of the connected world of global health governance, we would also have to be sure that de-escalation was not simply for a particular threat but that it did not compromise our ability to respond to public health threats in future. There's no use borrowing from Peter to pay Paul in public health; stopping one outbreak at the cost of all future outbreaks is not de-escalation in any sense when dealing with the so-called ultimate bioterrorist.

Two cases illustrate this. In the first, failure of de-escalation is proximate. We might think of a jurisdiction whose emergency powers include eminent domain if contaminated structures needed to be destroyed in an emergency.[25] We could imagine a situation in which an environment thought to harbor animals that are vectors for a dangerous pathogen is destroyed. A predictable result of this is the displacement of just those animals, potentially into towns. The public health measure is both preventative because there's no imminent threat, but it is also self-defeating: it drives the carriers of the emerging threat into other locations and makes them harder to deal with in future. There may be ways to slowly remove this threat through other means such as catch and release, selective culling, or even animal vaccination programs.

A longer, more complex issue is the issue of vaccines. A small number of scholars have suggested vaccine mandates as a way to solve vaccine-preventable illnesses, especially with recent spikes in vaccine resistance and denial, and especially during pandemics that threaten to overwhelm health systems.[26] From the quasi-realist health security perspective, there seems to be an in-principle reason to do so: mandating vaccines would give better coverage, and would prevent the onset of pandemic diseases. One way to counter this might be to appeal to the ineffectiveness of mandates in nonsecuritized settings such as childhood vaccinations.[27] Yet a reason why this might fail, even if it were to be found to be effective in preventing the resurgence of a vaccine-preventable disease or an immediate pandemic, is that it would almost certainly undermine pandemic preparedness writ large. Vaccine resistance is driven, in no small part, by broader mistrust of government.[28] Trust is a resource and at times might be spent to gain something else. But there's no need to fetishize trust to see that increasing distrust through vaccine mandates will make it more difficult to secure trust at a later stage and will deplete a scarce resource that might be needed for coercive means during future public health emergencies. Broad vaccine mandates pursued by a public health authority absent just cause and in the absence of a sound public engagement project may seem attractive on their face, but they fail to satisfy basic "peacetime" public health ethics and make public health emergencies harder to declare and act on. There is a role for mandates, but it is not through the democratic and not through the emergency process.

There may be a role for liberty-limiting measures outside of a public health emergency. They, however, must be consistent with the principle of last resort, and further with a principle of de-escalation that bridges the gap between public health ethics outside an emergency, and within it. The aim must be to pull a community back from a potential crisis, and further not to endanger their future readiness against future emergencies. This is a demanding principle, but it is one that views liberty-limiting measures as part of a broader strategy of securing communities against infectious disease.

Conclusion: Balancing Principles

In this chapter, I described normative principles for the declaration of a public health emergency. This provides a scheme around which future or reformed emergency powers could be designed: a criterion for declaring emergencies and assessing the use of emergency declarations. It also completes our comparison between the classic *ad bellum* tenets of just war theory and resolves some outstanding issues with the orthodox view (table 6.2).

One outstanding issue here is the degree to which all these principles must be fulfilled for an emergency to be just. But merely fulfilling them all is not the end of the story. Recalling the previous chapter, it may be the case

Table 6.2
Correspondence between just war theory and public health ethics (update 2)

Temporal/contextual feature	Just war theory	Public health ethics
Before the crisis	Legitimate authority	Legitimate authority
	Last resort	Last resort
	Just cause	Just cause
	Right intention	-
	Reasonable chance of success	-
	Proportionality	Proportionality
During the crisis	Necessity	Effectiveness & necessity
	Proportionality	Proportionality
	Discrimination	Least infringement
	??	Public justification
Outside the crisis	Legitimate authority	Legitimate authority

that declaring an emergency is indeed a last resort, but a last resort borne of some political failing. Here, an emergency may still be unjust. But it is unjust in the sense that an emergency that is a last resort but disproportionately harmful, or was engaged in when other alternatives were plentiful, is not.

A strict consequentialist might say that it is not as bad: it is unclear here whether one thing can be less unjust than another if both are unjust. What can clearly be said is that they are different in that what we ought to do about those injustices will be qualitatively different.[29] Least worst choices in the moment can still, ultimately, be unjust. One particularly critical case is raised by Daniel Schwartz and others in the case of self-defense: responses that are unjust because we fail to adequately prepare for an expected threat in a way that provides us a way out other than our last resort.[30] While a full exploration of Schwartz's work is beyond the scope of this work, if its major conclusion is true, it would make one of the starkest failures of the realist model of modern health security. That is, health security avoids the broader, structural questions of preventing a pandemic that arguably would obviate the need for as many crisis declarations and use of emergency powers, and in doing so leads us into emergency declarations that need not happen.

Some outstanding issues must remain until later chapters. Importantly, detail is needed regarding the end of an emergency. How we reform our institutions to reflect this demanding account, moreover, will remain for the final chapter in which the larger political concerns around securitization must be returned to.

With this in mind, we can now turn to the ethics of liberty-limiting measures. Because this is the most developed part of the orthodox view, I will do less to develop these ideas individually as I have here. Rather, the purpose is to show that military ethics has important insights into how we might permissibly pursue liberty-limiting measures during health emergencies, and what scope of those measures can be justified.

7 The Ethics of Liberty-Limiting Measures

The orthodox view of public health ethics focuses on the ethics of specific public health interventions. Of particular interest to health security are "liberty-limiting measures," such as quarantine, mandatory vaccinations, curfews, civil commitments, and border closures.[1] While some have argued that the most extreme of these measures are antiquated and could plausibly be replaced by robust nonemergency public health,[2] liberty-limiting measures continue to be popular public health tools. If anything, over time states appear to have become more accustomed to dishing those measures out. I have already discussed how, in Australia during the COVID-19 outbreak, explicit curfews and restrictions on movement for the city of Melbourne were instituted using the police to enforce lockdowns. These limits exceeded the stay-at-home orders common to the United States (erroneously referred to as "lockdowns"), which rarely if ever escalated to being enforced with the force of law.[3] The Melbourne lockdowns were considerably more extreme: individuals were forbidden from traveling more than 5 kilometers (3.1 miles) from their homes except for approved purposes such as work in permitted industries or caregiving; were subject to an 8pm–5am curfew; and were forbidden visitors among other limitations; this applied not to a small group but to a city of 4.9 million.[4]

Arguably the most famous liberty-limiting attempt was the total closure of the 11-million-person city of Wuhan, the epicenter of the COVID-19 outbreak in humans.[5] Travel into and out of the province of Hubei, in which Wuhan is located, was also restricted to stop the spread of the virus to the rest of China and beyond. This particular strategy is concerning, in part because it exceeds the recommendations for handling the outbreak provided by WHO and set out by IHR, and thus raised questions about the role of international law in global health.[6]

This chapter examines what liberty-limiting measures look like as we think through a theory of just health security. Despite the flurry of war metaphors in the opening months of the pandemic, only one dealt with the unique features of military ethics and how they might play out if applied to public health in a global pandemic.[7] This is despite the legal and moral basis of armed conflict being considerably more developed, and considerably more ancient, than the ethics of public health.

In *in bello* considerations, we find the most tendentious and difficult question of military ethics: when an individual acting on behalf of the state can kill others. In this body of work lie the antecedents of the doctrines of necessity and proportionality that the orthodox view develops, albeit in a somewhat confused way. As I discussed earlier, there is death and misery on the line when we enact public health policies. Thus we have to think carefully about what kinds of responses are justified, and when, to particular kinds of threats.

In what follows, I first detail *in bello* considerations, and in particular how recent debates in military ethics have attempted to square international humanitarian law governing killing in war with human rights law. This is critical in marrying ongoing debates about global health governance and human rights with the theory of public health emergencies developed over the last few chapters.

I then turn, and take as a case example, the recent debate around social distancing in the COVID-19 pandemic as a means to explore the ethics of liberty-limiting measures. I choose this case as a methodological move because it seems, on the one hand, innocuous: COVID-19 is a public health emergency if ever there was one, and social distancing seems less invasive than other liberty-limiting measures like vaccine mandates or quarantine. I show how social distancing can be seriously liberty limiting, and by applying the previous work on harm and domination from the impersonal account of disease.

I then make the case for an ethical framework for liberty-limiting measures in public health emergencies that is on the one hand more expansive than the orthodox view on account of fewer criteria and greater latitude in accomplishing public health aims in an emergency; but more restrictive in terms of how it conceives of obligations toward citizens caught up in pandemic response. I do this through a reading of the criteria for *jus in bello* that clarifies necessity, proportionality, and discrimination principles as they apply to public health.

I conclude by linking ethical considerations within public health emergencies to those outside emergencies. I argue that the liability the necessity principle sets up for states requires them to prepare not just during, but before the onset of emergencies to support citizens in pandemic response. This entails practical ethical considerations for how we make plans about technology, staff, and healthcare funding, resolve the aftermath of health emergencies, and engage in global governance.

Jus in Bello

Where *jus ad bellum* deals with the ethics of declaring war, *jus in bello* deals with the conduct of war itself. War can cause an almost incomprehensible amount of suffering. As such, an enormous body of literature deals with the ethics of armed conflict, international humanitarian law, and its intersection, with an eye toward the limits placed on suffering inflicted in the pursuit of war.

In general, there are three components to the ethics of conduct in war, compared to five of the orthodox view of public health ethics. The most critical of these is the principle of discrimination. This strongly demarcates combatants from noncombatants: civilians, the sick, the wounded, and humanitarian and aid groups in a war zone. The principle of discrimination prohibits the intentional targeting of civilians or civilian buildings as part of military operations, and holds that it is always worse to kill noncombatants than combatants.[8]

Next are necessity and proportionality. Military acts in war are permissible to the degree they are necessary to the objective of winning: ending war and restoring a lasting peace. This includes the killing of enemy combatants, and whether acts of war inflict suffering on the enemy unnecessary to the task at hand. Military acts, moreover, are only permissible to the degree that their benefits outweigh the harms caused by their enactment. Much like *ad bellum* considerations, *jus in bello* takes specific kinds of benefits and harms into consideration but does so around individual military actions rather than the war as a whole. And they are both justified along similar grounds: because harming individuals is always on its face wrong, it is not enough to have an absence of reasons not to harm someone—we must have a positive reason to do so.[9]

A number of internal debates in military ethics that seek to revise the basic tenets of just war theory are important to the analysis that comes next. First, there is debate about what kinds of costs must be incurred to prevent civilian harm. Especially in humanitarian interventions, say the defense of a people against a despotic government, there may be cases in which prolonging a war is worse for civilians than finishing it quickly, and provides a reason to impose additional risk on civilians so long as it is not excessive or greater than would be imposed by other tactics that may prolong the war.[10] However, there remain strong reasons for a state and soldiers to accept additional liability in order to ensure civilian lives are preserved in prosecuting a war.[11]

The second concerns what constitutes "necessity." Until recently, modern understanding of this principle was that acts satisfied this principle if they conformed to the overall aims of military action. This was a broad understanding of necessity in which discretion played a large role: as long as an act was seen as contributing to military success, necessity was satisfied. Yet this interpretation has changed in recent years. Larry May, in particular, has argued that necessity should be viewed in considerably more strict terms than previously thought, and uses the evolution of international humanitarian law to demonstrate this. The International Committee of the Red Cross's 2009 *Interpretive Guidance on the Notion of Direct Participation in Hostilities under International Humanitarian Law* recommended that "the kind and degree of force which is permissible against persons not entitled to protection against direct attack must not exceed what is *actually* necessary to accomplish a legitimate military purpose in the prevailing circumstances." In 2013, they further claimed it would "defy basic notions of humanity to kill an adversary or to refrain from giving him or her an opportunity to surrender where there is manifestly no necessity for the use of lethal force."[12] While these two claims cut across each other in some ways, May has shown that both point to the idea that *actual* necessity is required, rather than a presumed or loose sense of necessity. That is, a clear operational connection is needed to the aim of restoring a lasting peace through the conflict. He further notes that while this is incredibly demanding of military commanders, it also supports a broadly contingent pacifist position that starts from true pacifism and then works back to a demanding position on war.[13]

This change arises in the context of harmonizing human rights law with humanitarian law in recent decades. In 2005, the High Court of Israel held that "a civilian taking part in direct hostilities cannot be attacked at such time as he is doing so, if a less harmful means can be employed." That is, civilians engaged in violent acts could not be engaged with lethal force unless actually necessary to protect citizens against imminent harm. This supports the 1996 International Court of Justice ruling against Israel that while civil and political rights might be temporarily overruled in time of national emergency, the right to life, and to not be deprived arbitrarily of one's life is non-derogable.[14] Both cases show increasing political consensus that human rights are not set aside during conflict, but rather must be consonant with conduct in war except in cases where there is genuine necessity on which the pursuit of the resolution of war depends.

A final controversy that is important for our discussion is the permissibility of killing in war and its relation to the declaration of war. Just war theory in its modern formulation holds that *ad bellum* and *in bello* considerations are independent. That is, unjust wars can be fought justly, and just wars can be fought unjustly. Recent work has challenged this, holding that unjust wars cannot be fought justly in principle, and that soldiers on an unjust side are liable to be killed where soldiers on the just side are not.[15]

The debate about revisionism in just war theory bears directly on health security, but with an important twist. In war, a sovereign nation has broken the peace, whereas the threat in a public health emergency, as in chapter 4, is primarily concerned with a response to a communicable disease. As one side—and typically the aggressor—is non-agential in virtue of being a virus, bacterium, fungus, or so on, questions of their liability to attack are not important. What is important is the general public during a public health emergency. Citizens not engaged in the institutional response to a public health emergency are, on this account, analogous to noncombatants. Their rights might be infringed upon in some cases, but only with a special justification. And the state ought to bear a cost in order to prevent those rights violations to begin with. The question, then, is: what cost? To understand that we turn to social distancing.

Social Distancing

Social distancing is a term that exploded into the lexicon in 2020, but as a series of practices the use of measures that change the spatial and temporal dimensions of communities to influence how infectious diseases spread has a long history. Frederick Law Olmsted, whose best-known work is New York's Central Park, described the park as "the lungs of the city," where individuals could inhabit open green space away from the crush of the rest of the city. While grounded in miasma theory, Olmsted's intuition is a testament to basic ideas of social distancing—that increasing the space between inhabitants of a community can reduce the spread of disease.[16] Similar effects can be found in the influence of tuberculosis on modernist architecture and public housing.[17]

Yet the term "social distancing" is not as well defined as other public health measures. While "quarantine" and "isolation" refer to the confinement of individuals who are suspected to be exposed to an infectious disease, or are clinically ill with that disease, respectively,[18] social distancing is a single name for a very broad set of acts, policies, and institutional choices. All these choices have at their core the aim of reducing the frequency of contact between individuals that may lead to the transmission of infectious disease.

Consider four paradigm cases of acts that might plausibly constitute social distancing. The first is guidance to wear masks, which may come in general recommendations for all members of a community, or for subsets (those who are symptomatic, in service work, on public transit, and so forth) of a community. This measure seeks to reduce the frequency of close contacts resulting in transmission by reducing the number of contacts that count as "close"; that is, reducing the incidence in which any contact results in the spread of respiratory droplets between individuals.

Next, closures of businesses or schools are a paradigm case of social distancing. These are broader forms of social distancing and achieve their effect by reducing the incidence of contacts within mass gathering settings. Business and school activities are necessarily ones in which individuals come into close contact, exchange materials that might carry infectious disease particulates (e.g., anything that can carry fomites), and are sites in which a number of communities might interact around a shared location, such as a big-box department store that services a number of towns. An indirect effect of this closure might be to reduce the incentives people have to leave their homes in the first place, which has secondary effects such as reduced sidewalk traffic or public transit use.

Background policy decisions may count as *de facto* social distancing policies. Mandated paid time-off policies are heterogeneous across the world, and even those that are in place are varied in the amount of time they allow, under what circumstances, and for what category of worker. Nonetheless, paid time-off policies have been associated with up to 40 percent reductions in seasonal influenza cases, and thus an important platform policy to encourage social distancing during an infectious disease outbreak, especially among healthcare workers and other groups vulnerable to infection.[19] In virtue of breaking transmission, therefore, it could count as a kind of social distancing measure.

Finally, the architectural and landscape decisions by cities and even nations can count as social distancing if they are designed to reduce the transmission of infectious disease. While these can be background conditions to how cities or nations endure an infectious disease outbreak, they can also be choices made during particular outbreaks, such as the city of Bogotá's decision to open forty-seven miles of temporary bike lanes to improve air quality and reduce crowding on public transport during the COVID-19 outbreak.[20]

These cases allow us first to distinguish between practices that seek to reduce the number of potentially transmission-causing interactions that occur, and those practices that seek to reduce the conditional probability, given an interaction, that transmission will occur. Second, we can distinguish between public health policies or practices that are individually performed, and those that are performed by organizations or social institutions. Third, we can distinguish between policies and practices that maintain social distancing regardless of whether a public health emergency arises, and those that are implemented within (and perhaps only within) a public health emergency.

The COVID-19 outbreak demonstrates how diverse these practices can be. Across the globe a range of measures have been enacted, with different levels of severity, to prevent the transmission of COVID-19.[21] These include stay-at-home orders, bans on large gatherings, business closures or seating limits, school closures, mask mandates, cancellations of elective surgeries, and prohibition of visitors in care facilities. In addition to national variation, some vary their policies by substate region, restricting social distancing measures only to those regions that have the highest number of cases.

This diversity offers an opportunity, by examining social distancing as a class of practice, to think critically about the kind of burdens these different practices might impose on individuals and communities during pandemics, and thus the conditions under which different practices are permissible. In particular, it offers a view of social distancing that sees it as, at times, a considerably invasive public health practice, but is in principle able to be designed in ways that mitigates some or even all of the infringements posed.

Interference and Domination

A chief reason to consider social distancing, rather than, say, quarantine, is as follows: where quarantine is often seen as a straightforwardly liberty-limiting practice,[22] social distancing is somewhat more opaque. A preliminary concern is if this is really an issue. But an advantage to resolving this question in the positive is that it can give us an insight into what should be expected of liberty-limiting actions in terms of satisfying the demands of just health security.

As a preliminary move, I set aside certain questions of effectiveness of social distancing measures. These have been answered to varying degrees elsewhere,[23] but there is a considerable amount of normative work to be done even once we have established the expected effectiveness of social distancing measures. Rather, I wish to inquire whether, as a matter of moral theory, these are the kinds of acts we should be concerned about in a theory of just health security.

The first concern to address is whether social distancing measures are liberty limiting in the first place. Part of the uncertainty here comes from the breadth of the term. It is questionable if measures involving paid time off, whether enacted on an emergency or normal legislative basis, or of urban design, or of indoor versus outdoor dining, are liberty limiting in any substantive sense. Still other measures may be subject to reasonable disagreement. Take business closures. One might claim a business owner's liberty is infringed upon if they have a right to run their business in the first place, but that the state may have a compelling interest to enforce such a closure in the name of public health. It is less straightforward to claim that a *consumer's* liberty is infringed upon, much less by the state, if such closures arise. This can be seen most starkly when closures are voluntary or in response to guidance over mandates: when the state of Georgia "reopened" from stay-at-home orders in April 2020, some business owners elected to keep their businesses shut.[24] It is not clear that consumers, or employees, have their liberty violated any more than if violated by businesses that remain closed on Sunday. It is also not immediately clear that employees had their liberty violated, any more than they have their liberties violated by not being able to work for their employers on Sunday. But I countenance that there may be some significant difference for a consumer's liberty rights between a store voluntarily closing due to a pandemic, either because of their own beliefs or in response to a public health agency's nonbinding recommendation, than if the shop is compelled to close by force of law.

The value at stake here is, I take it, liberty claims grounded in a voluntaristic, negative conception of liberty as noninterference. This is the sense used by the orthodox view, as Childress and Bernheim suggest, in thinking about what the authors of the orthodox view refer to as moral interests.[25] This conception of liberty is a strong presumption against direct interference in one's action by state power.

Yet I think this fails to capture two important senses in which social distancing measures can infringe upon liberty, albeit in less obvious ways. To understand, we can call upon the work up to the impersonal account of disease. Applied broadly enough, and for long enough, social distancing can damage our ability to form communities, and limit our opportunities in important ways. Freedom of movement and freedom of association are typically thought of in noninterference terms, such as when they are infringed upon through quarantine actions.[26] But the restrictions placed on individuals during social distancing can be conceived of in other terms, namely those that conceive of liberty as an exercise in nondomination.

Nondomination conceives of our rights not merely as the absence of interference in our activities, but in certain important assurances that those actions cannot be restricted in arbitrary and/or sudden ways. In particular, having such a right entails that you are generally free from some interference in making some sort of choice under certain circumstances; that those choices and circumstances are publicly salient and not at the mercy of the definitional sophistry of others; that you have a basis for believing you reliably enjoy this kind of freedom; and recourse if interference does occur.[27]

Unlike quarantine, in which individual freedoms are infringed upon in the obvious, noninterference sense and where that limitation is part of what quarantine entails, broader social distancing measures infringe on liberties in a slightly different way. They do this by infringing upon liberties as nondomination, disrupting life plans and breaking up communities—frequently arbitrarily. They do this, moreover, in ways that are frequently exogenous to the practice of social distancing, where the limitations could be lessened or even obviated through supportive measures. Not everyone is dominated in the same way, or even at all, by some social distancing measures. Working from home is considerably easier for some than others. Technology, especially in 2022, mediates the harms and benefits of social distancing. And so it is partly the way that our social distancing measures are structured, tactically, that determines their harms.

This takes us to the next concern: a belief about social distancing measures is that their benefits frequently outweigh their harms, at least in cases of serious harms. The ongoing tragedy of COVID-19 seems to make this obvious, but we should carefully think through why that is. There are two axes on which harms could arise. These axes are first, whether harm is directly or indirectly a result of some social distancing measure; and second, whether those harms are proximate/short-term, or ultimate/long-term. These are logically independent, as we see below.

Direct and proximate harms arise because social distancing is hurting an individual in the here and now. A paradigm example of direct, proximate harms arising because of social distancing are individuals who can't access nonpandemic (in this case, non-COVID-19) medical care as a result of social distancing measures. This may occur because an individual cannot access routine acute care services because of social distancing; because offices are closed, not accepting new patients, are no longer accessible for patients with disabilities, have inadequate telemedicine services for patients' needs, or must close because they lack sufficient personal protective equipment to operate safely.[28] Here, the distancing itself causes harm.

But direct, proximate harms from social distancing are surely more widespread than this. Any individual who is dominated in the sense I described above may also be harmed by social distancing if that domination prevents them from avoiding harm.[29] This includes, for example, individuals who are now confined with abusive family members (including family members they *discover* are abusive in the context of a protracted stay-at-home order) for an extended period, and are unable to access shelters or simply leave the house for some other safe location. A parallel epidemic of domestic violence worldwide has tracked the implementation of social distancing measures and the shuttering of social services in response to COVID-19. Both a lack of social services and increased financial insecurity of inappropriately enacted pandemic responses disproportionately affect women, particularly those who are acutely vulnerable to violence.[30]

Some individuals are indirectly and proximately harmed by social distancing arrangements right now. These include "essential personnel" expected to be physically present at their job in order to maintain community functions. Essential personnel are harmed indirectly by virtue of being required, perhaps under the threat of job loss, to be present at their work despite the additional risk. Obviously, this is sometimes justified and even required, such as healthcare workers. However, not all essential workers are essential in a justified sense. The US meat industry has continued during the pandemic as an "essential business," costing the lives of workers who are often vulnerable by virtue of poor working conditions, immigration status, and low wages.[31] We might take this two ways: either that the meat industry is not essential *simpliciter*, or that the meat industry is not so necessary that it shouldn't accept reduced productivity by incorporating appropriate social distancing measures within its activities to ensure worker safety. I leave aside which sense is true; in either case, this kind of harm arises because a particular social distancing measure or plan fails to protect individuals, and they may be injured or die as a result.

Individuals may be directly harmed by social distancing, but in a delayed fashion. Consider, for example, elective procedures or screening that may be put off by weeks or months as hospitals and medical centers seek to reduce appointments in order to prevent transmission of disease within their facilities. This raises a complex risk-benefit calculus: on the one hand, nosocomial transmission of COVID-19 is a definite risk; on the other, failure to conduct sufficient early screening for cancers, or perform preventative surgeries such as the removal of high-risk lesions, may cause delays in diagnosis that ultimately result in excess morbidity and mortality.[32] These individuals—and other individuals who are delayed in receiving diagnosis or treatment for some future risk—may not die for some time, but they may die sooner than otherwise because of social distancing measures today.

Finally, there are people who are indirectly harmed by social distancing over a long period. In addition to immediate financial harms to individuals as a result of social distancing practices, for example, there will be an aggregate toll that arises as folks caught up in long-term unemployment will be harmed. Recall that at its height, global unemployment was 9 percent, but considerably more for service workers, young people, people of color, women, and people with disabilities. This is an "actual cause of death," in the sense McGinnis and Feoge would use it,[33] where the absolute and relative employment discrepancies are the cause of mortality. Those who suffer the most deprivation under social distancing, even if they ultimately survive this pandemic, may borrow against the end of their life to weather the current storm.[34] We have not begun to see, I suspect, this kind of harm because the pandemic is still too close.

None of these harms is trivial, and many are lethal. These harms often arise, moreover, at sites of existing structural injustice. These are the "collateral damage" of public health. Lack of access to healthcare, weak employment rights, or having to congregate in settings in which sufficient protections from infectious disease are already lacking, undocumented immigrant labor, job insecurity, and poverty are all areas where the weapons we use against COVID-19 disproportionately harm citizens. They are nontrivial harms, often inflicted on the already marginalized and vulnerable.[35] And like the public health crisis they stem from, but harder to track, they accrue to populations.

Revised Criteria

Social distancing is thus not a mere inconvenience but can be a substantial violation of liberty. It is not harmless, and at times can even be fatal. How then, should we understand the permissibility of social distancing under just health security?

Let's start by going back to the orthodox view. The canonical example used in that work is surveillance. In that paper, the authors argue for the necessity of surveillance, but take the least infringement condition to do work in setting the scope of that surveillance, including whether it is active mandatory screening, active reporting from voluntary screening, or voluntary reporting and screening. The least infringement condition of the orthodox view, according to recent work by Allen and Selgelid, applies best when comparing measures that seek to accomplish the same subgoal in a public health strategy.[36] That is, where two or more measures accomplish the same subgoal, the least infringing measure ought to be used. Infringement, here, is taken broadly and not just in terms of liberty interests; so if opportunities can be preserved in enacting some public measure, they ought to be just so that the public health subgoal is preserved between these measures.

But I think just health security can do more than the orthodox view and replace the least restrictive means criteria with a more robust theory of action. Revising the *in bello* discrimination principle for public health, we can claim that human rights retain their force under a state of crisis: there is no *lex specialis*, or law governing a specific subject matter, of public health. This does not mean all liberty-limiting measures are perforce impermissible. Rather, we should resist them, and the actors that pursue these public health goals—in particular, the state—should accept liability in cases where these means become necessary to minimize their harms.

In the previous chapter I noted that proportionality and last resort were related in declaring a public health emergency because proportionality helps define the set of options over which we commit to a last resort. So too, proportionality and discrimination are related within a public health emergency. A revised discrimination version of the principle for health security holds

> *Discrimination*: the public should be spared harm or infringements on liberty when possible, and the state and its representatives have an obligation to accept the costs of sparing them that harm.

That means that, in a choice between alternative measures or different instantiations of measures combined with supportive measures, we should choose the option that least harms, dominates, or interferes with the liberty of individuals, and the state should accept significant liability for this action. These supportive measures may be, among others: compensatory such as replacing lost income; legal, in protecting individuals from eviction; or material, such as providing housing and food for citizens confined during lockdown. But the liability rests with the state, as the foundation of public health and the permissible use of force to enforce that health during an emergency. When the state does not implement these measures, it is acting unjustly. And importantly, it acts unjustly even if the means are proportionate and effective.

To understand why, consider that war allows for an extreme liberty-limiting measure—killing. However, it does not always allow for killing, and in particular when doing so would violate the rights of noncombatants. This is because noncombatants have not given up their rights in virtue of becoming threats that are liable to harm. But the story does not end there, because sometimes we perform acts in the pursuit of the just ends of war that do put civilians in harm's way. And it is always better to act in a way that imposes less risk when engaging in violent acts, then it is more risk. Seth Lazar, in his work on sparing civilians, gives us an argument as to why:

1. Endangerment is wrong, even if the risks imposed do not lead to harm;

2. Endangerment that violates a right, even if it could lead to harm but does not, is still a violation of that right;

3. If 1 and 2 are correct for any kind of harm, then they are also true when someone is exposed to *wrongful* harm because another intends to act in a way that causes them harm.[37]

Lazar explains that what grounds these is that endangerment constitutes a loss of security, understood as the avoidance of unchosen risks and wrongful harm. This is intrinsically valuable, but it is also deeply instrumentally valuable to planning our lives and enjoying other goods. When I endanger you, even if I do not harm you, I cause you stress and anxiety; but I also may disrupt your ability to plan for the future.[38] Here then, acts that impose risks of harms, including those from domination, are worse when they are riskier than if they are not. From the perspective of health security, we act unjustly when we impose additional risks on those we subject to public health actions, and we are liable for the burden of preventing those additional risks.

Having considered the proportionality and discrimination conditions, what of necessity? The orthodox view holds that public health interventions are justified, all other things being equal, if they are effective and necessary to accomplish some public health goal. But under just health security, that criterion is strengthened. Necessity instead points to goals of a public health emergency that would see its resolution. It is thus not sufficient that a liberty-limiting measure promotes the public's health. It must instead be established that it promotes public health in a way that is operationally linked to the ending of the public health emergency, or in de-escalating the chance of an expected public health crisis in the *ad vim* case, where we act to prevent a future crisis. Some measures may help, but not in the right way: they may improve public health but get us no closer to the end of the emergency. Alternately, some may be overdetermined, such as when a public health actor may be guilty of throwing in the kitchen sink in the absence of a coherent public health strategy designed to resolve the emergency. But the reason why we have license in the first place to perform these public health acts is the emergency itself, and so our actions must be laser focused to ending it.

Taken together, this provides us with two insights into public health action. A strong principle of necessity may provide us with greater latitude to act than the weaker principle hinted at by the orthodox view. If the aim of a public health emergency is to end the threat of a particular infectious disease, then lockdowns may be strongly necessary to achieve that aim, where a voluntary stay-at-home order is only weakly necessary to lower mortality but without ending the crisis. This means that even if the lockdown incurs greater harms or presents a greater rights infringement, it may be permissible just in case it satisfies an appropriate reading of the necessity condition where half measures do not. Put another way: there is no point in pursuing the proper aims of a justly declared public health emergency with half measures. If there is a positive reason to declare an emergency and act in a liberty-limiting way, then we should take measures that are necessary to fulfill that reason, and not some other reason (or no positive reason at all).

Second, replacing the least infringing measure criterion with a principle of discrimination entails that the state ought to incur significant liability for avoiding harms, including violations of liberty, on the public. This is not just a matter of proportionality, but because taking supportive measures that reduce risk respects agents as ends in themselves and promotes their personal security. This is true even if the person in question would not have ultimately been harmed by the risks we impose upon them.

What of public justification? Three answers are available to us here. The first is that the public has a right to engage in deliberations about liberty-limiting measures in proportion to their bargaining power, as under Moehler's scheme described in previous chapters. But public justification also forms part of a scheme of nondomination, where informing and involving the citizenry about public health measures before they need to be used is part of securing the relevant options to act in a nonarbitrarily restricted way. It also meets Lazar's criteria grounded in security, where it enables individuals to make sufficient revisions to their life plans consistent with a necessary public health action. This places the emphasis on public justification, importantly not just within a public health emergency, but preceding it.[39] Despite the prevalence of editorials and opinion pieces claiming we are "not ready for the next pandemic,"[40] what was almost never done in practice was the process of actually preparing individuals on whom risk would be imposed on a day-to-day basis for what the next pandemic would entail.

Finally, and perhaps inhering closest to the war metaphor, is the idea of hearts and minds. It has, for thousands of years, been an integral part of strategy that if you lay the moral ground of a people properly, then you will never have cause to war with them.[41] Public justification gives rise to the possibility of a public that is cooperative and even enthusiastic about resisting a public health threat. Without it, the public will sour, and the battle becomes not just against the virus but a people who do not understand and even resent an imposition that diminishes their lives any way the dice fall. A just health security begins with communication as a strategy with which to create options for public health, and not as an afterthought once we know what we want to do.

Evaluating Social Distancing Measures

How then, should we evaluate the ethics of different social distancing measures? Here, I describe three strategies for doing so. These strategies are not mutually exclusive, and there are reasons to engage in each. Importantly, they accomplish different goals. First and perhaps most obviously, we can evaluate social distancing measures in a decision-theoretic sense. That is, for proposed or enacted social distancing measures, we can ask: to what extent do these social distancing measures satisfy our ethical criteria?

There are a number of plans for enacting, continuing, and lifting social distancing measures we could evaluate here. It is not the purpose of my book to comprehensively evaluate all proposed measures, but some illustrative examples will help. The National Governors Association in 2020 listed seven major reports that contain recommendations for public health readiness and reopening, of which five explicitly addressed social distancing.[42] Of those five, however, only two addressed supportive measures during social distancing that may enhance opportunities or reduce the harms of social distancing on those subject to it, with mixed results. Vital Strategies' "Box It In" noted the essential nature of providing services and support to people under quarantine so that they will better adhere to quarantine requirements. This is consistent with CDC SARS recommendations for quarantine,[43] but Vital Strategies appears to be broader in its scope in virtue of its opening claim that "Although almost all of the U.S. population has been asked to shelter in place and otherwise observe physical distancing, compliance varies greatly among communities, illustrating challenges adhering to quarantine."[44] It is not clear, however, the degree to which Vital Strategies is committed to broader social supports during social distancing, or only for quarantine; that is, of individuals believed to be exposed to COVID-19, which does not describe most individuals under social distancing.

The report by Allen and colleagues for the Edmond J. Safra Center for Ethics at Harvard University, on the other hand, accounted for the infringement associated with social distancing. While the report's use of "supported isolation" including healthcare and financial supports only referred to essential personnel, it did so in two important ways. First, it proposed an expanded essential workforce as part of a large-scale mobilization, particularly in contact tracing, that sought to retrain workers for tasks pertaining to pandemic response. Second, it sought to use supported isolation not as a supplement to, but as a replacement for widespread collective quarantine as a method of disease control[45]—that is, it sought to limit the infringement on the public by focusing on a large-scale mobilization of resources, replacing what had been termed the suppression model of control with a containment model.[46]

So, of five high-level reports that deal with social distancing, it appears only two came close to interrogating how these measures could plausibly be designed to mitigate the infringement on individual liberties in the relevant sense; only one went so far as to suggest a (partial) ordering of how these measures ought to be undertaken. None, however, addressed the required social, educational, financial, and medical support needed if extreme social distancing measures were required—which they were. This is partial evidence that the majority of reports favored at a high level by governments and public health authorities would not satisfy the demands of just health security insofar as they deal with ranking and selecting the appropriate social distancing measures.

The second way we can evaluate social distancing measures is by assessing, often retrospectively, how they perform. Elsewhere, I have argued that the ethics of responses to biological disasters, including pandemics, can be evaluated in terms of how we prepare for, act during, and respond after a disaster.[47] We can do the same when we consider social distancing measures. Here, moreover, we can evaluate the suite of social distancing measures taken together and individually. This has been done in a preliminary fashion in empirical terms for a number of countries.[48] An open question remains about whether we should evaluate social distancing measures for their permissibility based on all three components taken together, or each separately. There are strong reasons to think that if the justification for some act rests on a number of separate justificatory components, then failing in one entails failing to justly/permissibly enact the measure altogether.[49] This mirrors ongoing discussions in the ethics of war, about whether it makes sense to separate out the justness of a war's declaration, pursuit, and after-math; or whether a war is only just if those three elements are all just.[50] This is a demanding standard but—if we are engaged in retrospective analysis of social distancing measures—will identify how, or how badly we failed to achieve our goals in meeting the standards of ethics during a pandemic.

The final way we could evaluate social distancing measures is by deter-mining whether and how our basic institutions can satisfy our ethical standards in terms of social distancing. That is, we can ask how should our healthcare, education, economic, and other institutions be designed to deal with events such as pandemic disease. In evaluating the Repub-lic of Korea's approach to COVID-19, for example, a consistent message is that the nation's experience with Middle Eastern respiratory syndrome coronavirus demonstrated important weaknesses in the country's capabili-ties to respond to the arrival of a novel infectious agent. The reason the Republic of Korea has succeeded to a greater degree than the US, and thus has adopted far less invasive and liberty-infringing social distancing mea-sures, is partly in virtue of their institutions being prepared to respond to infectious disease.[51] Public health ethics can thus evaluate social distanc-ing in terms of the structure of basic institutions as capable or incapable of responding to infectious disease in a proportionate, effective, necessary, minimally infringing, and publicly justifiable way.

Just Health Security: Flexible but Demanding

This revised set of principles is flexible but demanding, more so than the orthodox view. It is flexible because it takes the state of a public health emergency as something we should resolve as quickly as possible, for the good of a community. And so it may allow for more stringent measures than the orthodox view just in case those measures are likely to be effective in ending a public health emergency. This is an extreme mandate, and may justify expansive powers.[52] However, it is extreme in the context of what, as discussed in the last chapter, a public health emergency is, and (as I discuss in chapter 9) what constitutes the end of an emergency.

However, the doctrine is also more demanding. It is demanding first because I have claimed that what it means for a liberty-limiting measure to be necessary is one that is *strongly* necessary to achieve the resolution of a public health emergency. This is considerably more demanding than the standard provided by the orthodox view.

This doctrine is also more demanding because it places considerable burden on the state to select measures that reduce the risk or infringement on individuals at considerable liability to itself. It is not sufficient to institute a stay-at-home order if the order could be paired with a basic subsistence package and guarantee of housing. These are not optional extras to a public health response under just health security, any more than checking a building is free of civilians before throwing a grenade into it is an optional extra for soldiers. Failing to do so turns liberty-limiting measures into a form of collective punishment, a violation of individual rights, and a failure to respect individuals as agents (table 7.1).

One obvious objection is, why not just lock down a country every time? The answer to this is threefold. The first is that not all public health threats rise to the level of a public health emergency and using such a measure outside of responding to the kind of threat that invokes a declaration of one would likely escalate into a breakdown of the public state. The second is that even within a public health emergency it isn't always necessary to end the emergency through a large-scale lockdown when a small lockdown will do; or use some other measure entirely. Contact tracing and isolation, appropriately financed and carefully conducted, for example, are still by and large the best measures in public health. The third is that a repeat strong lockdown strategy is unlikely to be consented to under the state I envisaged in

Table 7.1

Comparison between just war theory and just health security (update 3)

Temporal/contextual feature	Just war theory	Public health ethics
Before the crisis	Legitimate authority	Legitimate authority
	Last resort	Last resort
	Just cause	Reasonable aim
	Right intention	-
	Reasonable chance of success	-
	Proportionality	Proportionality
During the crisis	Necessity	Necessity
	Proportionality	Proportionality
	Discrimination	Discrimination

chapter 5, by citizens within the negotiating power they actually have. We have already seen this in COVID-19 as nations that once had control of the outbreak unravel as the global pandemic shows no signs of slowing.

Conclusion

In this chapter I covered the ethics of public health measures within a public health emergency. The principles of just health security, applied seriously, provide us with two novel findings. The first is that necessity may in fact demand more from us in aid of quickly resolving a public health emergency than the orthodox view admits. The second is that the demandingness of proportionality and discrimination criteria applied to public health mean that states are on the hook for considerably more resources in order to justify liberty-limiting measures. This follows from the strong interplay between human rights and the special regime of the emergency we have constructed.

This concludes the section of the book that deals with the two primary arms of classical just war theory and reconciles public health ethics with the normative structure it parallels. It provides a security-apt account of public health ethics that doesn't deny the relevance of securitization theory or criticisms of the orthodox view, but rather takes them as the starting point from which a coherent view of the ethics of public health security must derive.

The last two chapters extend insights from military ethics into less discussed, but still important aspects of the ethics of health security.

8   Drawing up the Troops: Waging War on Disease

The *Time* Person of the Year for 2014 was not one person, but a group: the "Ebola Fighters," the many healthcare workers active in Liberia, Guinea, and Sierra Leone. The article closed with one of those classic war metaphors:

> Early in the epidemic, CDC director Frieden spoke of Ebola's "fog of war." Its shroud covers the battlefield. Eventually—though no one can say when—the Ebola fighters are going to be victorious. The fog will clear, leaving the hard truth in view: this won't be the last epidemic. And when the next one comes, the world must learn the lessons of this one: Be better prepared, less fearful, less reactive. Run toward the fire and put it out together. Even more important, though, when the next one comes, remember the Ebola fighters and hope that we see their like again.[1]

The work of healthcare workers is tireless and potentially risky at the best of times, but during a crisis that burden is impossible to sustain long term. Public health emergencies allowed to go on will inevitably deplete healthcare workers of their energy, their time, and their concentration; eventually, it can and does kill them. During the 2013–2016 Ebola virus disease outbreak, the already fragile Liberia lost 8 percent of its healthcare workers to the virus.[2] Healthcare workers are perhaps the most precious and scarce resource in a pandemic. Their experience and training takes years or even decades to replace, and yet they are routinely ignored as a vulnerable and scarce resource during a pandemic.[3]

This chapter is about the people of pandemics. It might seem that here, the securitization of health breaks down most completely. This is because healthcare workers and soldiers are not at all the same. They are not trained the same; they do not have the same social and institutional structure or serve similar ends. Nonetheless, an account of just health security, drawing from military ethics, can teach us a few things.

In what follows, I apply the insights from the impersonal account of disease, and of last resort and liberty-limiting measures, to healthcare workers. After a brief comment on "essential personnel," I argue that under just health security, an emergency response that unduly jeopardizes healthcare workers is unjust. This injustice conflicts with the individual fiduciary duties healthcare workers possess to those under their care, who—unlike soldiers with those they fight—have strong positive reasons to provide care. The people they protect, however, may at times be hostile to them. Keeping to the method of this book, I frame this as an ethical and political-philosophical problem and discuss the institutional role that needs to be played to protect healthcare worker safety. Healthcare workers may be heroes, as Frieden suggests—but heroes often exist because leaders fail us.

I turn then to the role of those *leaders* in public health. I note that much like military strategy on securing cooperation (e.g., "winning hearts and minds") requires leadership, public health authorities also need to be vested with a certain kind of leadership. This leadership, I argue, has a normative ethical component to it that suggests what leaders ought to be and how they ought to behave. I conclude with an example, again from COVID-19, that demonstrates how the state as legitimate authority and the ethics of leadership can fail in public health, as a way to solidify the claim about their importance.

"Essential Personnel"

Before continuing, two more clarifications are required, particularly in terms of the current outbreak. The first concerns "essential personnel." When we discuss essential personnel in medical ethics, we typically have physicians, or more broadly healthcare workers in mind.[4] These are essential in the sense that without them, clinical care for individuals suffering from COVID-19 would not happen. We are concerned about these personnel in terms of the continuing functioning of the healthcare system.

Contrast this with "essential businesses," including those found in government ordinances around COVID-19.[5] What constitutes "essential" here is considerably broader than simply healthcare organizations. It certainly includes basic government services ("businesses" very broadly construed) including power and sanitation, but also employees at grocery stores and food service companies, law enforcement offices, scientists who need to engage in lab work as part of the outbreak response, lab techs who may need lab access to preserve samples even if experiments are halted, and so on. These are very broad categories and may vary from state to state.

This is significant, as what type and how many people in a population count as "essential" may impact the degree to which social distancing measures work or are justified. For example, on March 20, 2020, the US Undersecretary for Defense for Acquisition and Sustainment, Ellen Lord, released a memo declaring defense contractors essential personnel, and requiring them to continue to deliver products on time.[6] While some defense contractors may be engaged in essential work in the same way as healthcare workers, and indeed support them through the development of personal protective equipment or vaccines, others perform work far outside such a mandate. In cities and towns with large numbers of defense contractors whose work (truly essential or not) requires them to leave their homes, the population active and capable of transmitting COVID-19—and the population that therefore needs to support them in the form of transit workers, grocery store clerks, fast food workers, custodial staff, and more—will remain higher than in other locations.

I think that by and large, there is a sense in which "essential personnel" is a term that can be subject to reasonable disagreement. It can be based on substantive disagreements on what individuals and communities take to be essential; it could also potentially change based on the etiology of a particular disease or health crisis. What I take to be a core element of what makes someone essential personnel is that their continued work *in the setting in which they typically work* is necessary to maintain some kind of critical community function, or outbreak response. This includes clinical care, yes, but would include keeping the lights on, but also keeping people fed, properties from falling into disarray that may endanger community welfare, promoting rule of law, and scientific research aimed at resolving the crisis. Their essential role, moreover, typically means that in the context of the crisis they are exposed to some kind of risk in virtue of maintaining their role in its usual setting.

The content of "essential personnel" in a public health state becomes important because it broaches a question that my anthropologist colleagues might take on: "Essential for whom?" When we talk about the public health state, taking essential personnel to only be healthcare workers frames the role of state in providing a public health institution only in terms of its healthcare workforce. It may mean, for example, that the provision of masks to hospitals is seen as the only significant site of a public health masking campaign, rather than ensuring that service workers also get high-quality masks or respirators. Even within healthcare facilities, we might find that, as happened during the early stages of the COVID-19 pandemic, only the *clinical* healthcare workforce "counts" for mask allocation. This means that custodial staff at hospitals, who make take on extensive risky activities in cleaning and disinfecting rooms, may be denied masks because while they are genuinely essential to a response effort, they are not *counted* as essential, and thus not ensured the kind of protections we would otherwise think should be provided to these individuals.[7]

We can think of this as part of the justice of our emergency preparedness. If we are building a stockpile of equipment for our pandemic, we might decide that we need X masks, where X is defined as Y times the number of essential personnel, Z. What Z counts as, then, is of extreme importance, and has moral content. Failure to properly account for who contributes to essential roles in prosecuting a public health emergency means we have failed to prepare adequately. And failure to prepare adequately can mean that public health emergency declarations are not truly necessary (because we had other means at our disposal that we elected not to take), or that our actions are unjust within an emergency (because we fail to assume liability for protecting individuals from the harms of our public health actions when we could do otherwise).

Duty to Treat

Healthcare workers are frequently exposed to risks. At times, those risks are extreme. This has produced a literature on "duty to treat" in which bioethicists have asked whether, and under what conditions healthcare workers (but particularly physicians, arising from prejudices in the AIDS crisis) could refuse to treat infectious patients.[8] In general, the consensus has been that physicians do have a duty to treat, as do other healthcare workers, and that the duty to treat is quite strong. However, a lack of access to sufficient PPE and other safety equipment may arguably call this into question.[9]

What is asked less frequently is how these individual ethical decisions are bracketed by their social and political context. The decision to treat is not made in isolation. Writing in 1996, Leigh Turner asked of individuals arriving in critical care units with gunshot wounds "why do we not interrogate how they ended up here?"[10] This is particularly salient in a public health emergency, in which the degree to which patients arrive in a hospital over time reflects gaps in the capacities of public health to prevent illnesses from occurring. This does not place culpability for that risk on public health strictly—healthcare workers still have autonomy—but it does place healthcare workers at the most acute end of a series of decisions over which they may not have control.

Much like, it turns out, soldiers.

Traditionally, soldiers have been subject to what is known as the *unlimited liability thesis*, a doctrine that states that soldiers are expected to take on risks in the pursuit of the aims of war, including risks that will inevitably lead to their deaths.[11] This is a strong doctrine, and controversial for it. It is certain healthcare workers are not subject to unlimited liability, but recent debate about the thesis reveals how we might think about them in the context of public health emergencies.

The unlimited liability thesis in war has come into question. The consonance between human rights and international humanitarian law in the previous chapters. It follows that if soldiers do not forfeit their human rights by virtue of being soldiers, then their rights to life are not absolutely waived. They may be ordered to place themselves at risk, but that does not give commanders unlimited license with the lives of their troops. The principle of necessity should be respected in its strict form with one's own soldiers as well as noncombatants and enemies.[12]

This has important implications for healthcare workers when we view their liability through the lens of just health security. While healthcare workers have no human enemy under the impersonal account of disease, they still take on liability in their roles defending the public against this threat and in ways that respond to the rights of individuals under their care or on whom public health measures are imposed. They may care for acutely ill patients, patients' families, fill prescriptions, contact trace, conduct surveillance testing, administer vaccines, and so on. All of these can impose serious risk on a healthcare worker.

Healthcare workers thus take on considerable liability during public health emergencies. They do so in virtue of their professional role, serving in the fundamental social institution that is public health. But that liability ought not be unlimited. In particular, the state may act unjustly when it imposes upon healthcare workers significant but avoidable risks in the discharge of their duties. Like everyone else, healthcare workers engaged in the work of responding to a justly declared public health emergency have not waived their rights. Imposing significant extra risk on them violates their rights in the same way as I described in the previous chapter around liberty-limiting measures—it fails to respect their security and interests as persons. This is true in war, under international humanitarian law; so too is it true in public health. The public health state is not one that can condone the equivalent of Tennyson's description of British cavalry in the *Charge of the Light Brigade*:

> Theirs not to reason why,
> Theirs not to make reply,
> Theirs but to do and die.[13]

Two cases illustrate this case. The first are in cases of substandard personal protective equipment, a common feature of the COVID-19 pandemic. In cases where authorities cannot provide access to basic equipment, healthcare workers are jeopardized in ways not required of them by virtue of their professional role. When states fail to act on their obligations to bring an emergency to a close quickly and to limit the spread of disease with appropriate supports, they place healthcare workers at unnecessary risk. Healthcare workers are wronged to the degree that they are placed at greater than necessary risk of infectious disease where permissible alternate pathways to prevent the transmission of disease exist, and thus treating patients in an emergency can be limited. And to head off accusations that this is a case in which the government had no obligation because it was an unforeseen issue (a form of "ought implies can"), a projected lack of personal protective equipment has been a hallmark of the health security community that has dominated the policy landscape for decades, making it not just foreseeable but *foreseen*.[14]

The second case illustrates how we might expect (suitably attired, trained, and supported) healthcare workers to risk their lives in service of a public health goal. It is increasingly common that nations are turning to technological solutions to manage contact tracing. A plethora of contact tracing apps arose over the course of the COVID-19 pandemics but this technology was also pioneered, to considerable failure, during the 2013–2016 Ebola virus disease outbreak.[15] Yet these same episodes show that there is considerable evidence to suggest that contact tracing apps are less effective than older means.[16] Older means may be more costly; this is the role of the public health state. They may also be riskier because they require additional interaction with close contacts of infected individuals; this is the role of healthcare workers. Taking risks to ensure that contact tracing is done correctly, by going to local communities and engaging with them directly, exposes a healthcare worker to a higher chance of disease. But it is in the service of an arguably necessary component of a strategy to resolve a public health emergency.

This risk, however, should be imposed for a version of contact tracing that is necessary and expected to succeed in a crisis. What this ought to mean is not imposing greater risk on existing healthcare workers, but an obligation on behalf of states to recruit, train, and retain many more of them. This will mean maintaining larger volumes of public health workers on staff in local communities than currently exist. And like soldiers in war, it means maintaining sufficient numbers to rotate them off their duties as needed so they don't burn out or become so tired that they compromise the effectiveness of the mission; and give them work outside of a crisis so that their skills are maintained and they can be called up as needed. One of the key features of a modern military is that its soldiers spend the majority of their time not fighting wars. Public health can and should afford to be the same way. It is arguably justified under a public health state that takes seriously a principle of last resort—an early response involving contact tracing is rights preserving and even if activated as a partly securitized means is more likely to satisfy the principle of de-escalation than most other practices.

Public Health Leadership

The second kind of role I want to address is public health *leadership*. The role of leaders is almost totally understudied in public health ethics. This is a mistake, and it is significant that we have not individual but collections of moral accounts of physicians, police officers, and warfighters as leaders,[17] but none for public health officials. The study of public health leadership is also important given the political moment in which this book is written and the need for an *action guiding* account of public health ethics. Leadership is both understudied and in current public health often fragmented and weak as an institutional property. Those leaders that do exist, moreover, may lack the legitimacy or the authority to direct a public health response. This is a significant problem for the prospect of responding to public health needs. It is not to say those leaders that exist are not good leaders in principle; it is often that they do not occupy institutional roles that allow their leadership to be effective.

To illustrate this, consider the comments of the editorial board of the *New England Journal of Medicine* in October 2020:

> The response of our nation's leaders has been consistently inadequate. The federal government has largely abandoned disease control to the states. Governors have varied in their responses, not so much by party as by competence. But whatever their competence, governors do not have the tools that Washington controls. Instead of using those tools, the federal government has undermined them. The Centers for Disease Control and Prevention, which was the world's leading disease response organization, has been eviscerated and has suffered dramatic testing and policy failures. The National Institutes of Health have played a key role in vaccine development but have been excluded from much crucial government decision making. And the Food and Drug Administration has been shamefully politicized, appearing to respond to pressure from the administration rather than scientific evidence. Our current leaders have undercut trust in science and in government, causing damage that will certainly outlast them. Instead of relying on expertise, the administration has turned to uninformed "opinion leaders" and charlatans who obscure the truth and facilitate the promulgation of outright lies.[18]

This is a startling level of candor by a longtime medical institution such as the *New England Journal of Medicine*. It would not be the last: Holden Thorpe, editor in chief of *Science*, would in 2022 accuse the Biden administration of "sheepishly waving a checkered flag on the pandemic." He obliquely mentions leadership in closing:

> Legendary public health leader Paul Farmer summed up this situation well: "Those whose lives are rarely touched by structural violence are uniquely prone to recommend resignation as a response to it," he said. "In settings in which all of us are at risk, as is sometimes true of contagion shared through the air we breathe, we must also contemplate containment nihilism—the attitude that preventing contagion simply isn't worth it."[19]

Here, Thorpe invokes the late Paul Farmer, whose role in pandemics has been less official than that of a president or surgeon general, and more through his professional status and long career of excellence in the field of global health.

These examples provide a couple of useful distinctions. We can distinguish first between leadership as a character trait, and leadership as a role. The former is a set of properties that arise from an individual that makes them capable of effectively directing individuals to group action, including those skills that motivate people to act in coordinated ways. Good leaders can arise anywhere and need not occupy institutional roles. Students in group discussion can exercise good leadership, for example, in directing conversation even in the absence of an instructor's direction. Good leaders guide action, and model appropriate behavior and other positive group traits to their subordinates. Farmer held leadership roles at Harvard University and Brigham and Women's Hospital, but he also stood as a voice of authority in public health.

Leadership as a role is a property of institutions that function in a coordinating and action-guiding role over a collective action. Leadership can be more or less proximate, such as a leader of a unit in a government department, or an attending physician in a war in a hospital. At their most extreme they can be ultimate, such as a head of state or government. Leadership as a role is about guiding institutions or organizations to set aims and being held accountable for organizational failures. Anthony Fauci, as the director of the National Institute of Allergy and Infectious Diseases, occupies an institutional leadership position within that organization and within its parent organization, the National Institutes of Health. However, he does not occupy the kind of leadership position that, in the United States, would require confirmation of the Senate; nor does the National Institutes of Health hold a position within the executive branch of the United States that sets public health policy. Likewise, the chief medical officer of many countries is capable of advising government on public health, but has no leadership powers in the sense of executive control over a function of government.

Leadership in institutions is not necessarily a hierarchical role, though it can be and often is. Leaders need not always have higher levels of entitlements in an institution. Market theories of labor might suggest that leaders ought to have higher pay or more perks in order to attract the best candidates but it is never clear the degree to which this kind of incentive actually places good leaders in the right roles. It is plausible that the only thing that ultimately separates leaders from others is their coordination role.

Sometimes leadership roles are context specific. Military physicians, for example, may exercise leadership *qua* coordination and executive power in medical matters in the armed forces, but they have no power regarding strategic troop deployment. We could also envisage more radical institutional leadership dynamics, such as transient leadership roles for individual tasks such as the appointment of an *ad hoc* leader for a single task, or *de minimis* direction powers for a leader, such as the leadership of a traditional labor union in which a leader might have the capacity to prioritize or bring to order certain coordination activities, but direction on the ground is taken by members.

The traits and institutional roles of leaders come apart in important ways. Everyone has had the experience, I suspect, of interacting with someone in an institutional leadership role who is manifestly unfit to lead in terms of their character. We have also probably interacted with individuals who exercise strong leadership as a disposition but have no formal institutional role. It is possible that institutions sometimes serve their purpose even when corrupted or mismanaged by leaders because the latter exist to interpret, subvert, or act in spite of the former.

If leadership is an institutional role, however, it must be for the moral ends of the institution. In part, we judge institutional leaders and their actions in the context of their institution's purported ends, and the degree to which those ends are achieved. Organized criminal networks have leaders,[20] but those leaders are unethical in part because they are leading unethical organizations: they are directing an organization to immoral ends. Alternately, CEOs might lead companies, but a "moral CEO" may sound incongruous given that companies, in virtue of not being institutions guided by a moral purpose, have no moral ends. Leaders might be seen as compromised, even if acting within their means and in otherwise justified ways, if it is seen that the ultimate purpose of an institution has been compromised. I suspect that, for example, opponents of the US torture program will view leaders within US institutions that practice or did practice torture as compromised to the degree that the torture program represents a form of institutional corruption.[21]

The faces of leadership, good and bad, can be seen in the response to the COVID-19 outbreak. On the one hand, a common characterization of the diagnoses for the failure of states to respond adequately to the pandemic is a failure of leadership.[22] On the other hand, individuals who display leadership outside institutional roles have emerged as the public has turned to informal channels for education in an information-rich, knowledge-poor outbreak.

Still others have emerged and exhibited leadership despite occupying roles that are not appropriate for the purpose. Dr. Anthony Fauci emerged in the early days of the outbreak in the US as a clear voice of leadership and authority, owing in part to his previous role in the eventual US government response to the HIV/AIDS crisis. Fauci has no statutory authority, however, from which to coordinate and direct a public health response; Fauci's *de facto* leadership role was diminished following his removal from the White House Coronavirus Task Force under the Trump administration and then reelevated under the Biden administration. Nonetheless—and giving full credit to Fauci's dispositional leadership and coordination powers—it is unclear what leadership role the director of the National Institute for Allergy and Infectious Disease *should* take, now that Fauci has departed.

Fauci's role, and those of the various "czars" and taskforce heads in the US government, however, point to the lack of actual leadership displayed by those people who occupied formal *roles* in the US. President Trump, most infamously, was revealed by Bob Woodward in September of 2020 to have known of the seriousness of the pandemic but refused to act for his own reasons related to reelection.[23] To invoke securitized language, the commander in chief was caught in dereliction of his duty as a leader. Likewise, later reports from the CDC showed how leaders within that organization had been slowly divested of authority and corrupted away from their institutional roles by ordering subordinates to delete emails seeking to downplay COVID-19's risk to children.[24]

These are all examples of leadership troubles, but what is less explored is the fragmented and fundamentally weak leadership structure of American public health. Public health in America, unlike war in America, is not coordinated or directed in a way that even pretends to be grounded in reasons of any kind—moral or not. It, moreover, is one that has been eroded not just during the Trump administration, but over decades. Public health in the United States, after all, has its origins in military movements and the US Surgeon General's Office, which carries with it leadership of the United States Public Health Service Commissioned Corps. The surgeon general looks like a leadership office in the US if ever there was one.

Yet the surgeon general's office is a curious position. A full history of the office is provided by Stobbe, who describes its beginnings as a coordinating role in managing Naval quarantine hospitals.[25] But over time, the surgeon general's position was subsumed into the larger portfolio of what is now the Department of Health and Human Services. Caught between the larger political office of the department, and the power of the National Institutes of Health within that agency (and which Stobbe identifies as a historic enemy of the field of public health), the office was ultimately neutered by successive secretaries until it reached its present form, which is more a public relations office than a leadership position in the coordination sense I identified above. This leaves a public health system stranded between a massive and internally fragmented department, state agencies, local authorities, and the president, with occasional input from the National Security Council. While the US Department of Defense is hardly a streamlined organization, the US public health system is positively broken in comparison.

The discussion of leadership has been rehearsed recently in Australia, regarding state and federal leadership positions. Across states, the powers of state chief medical officers differ. In the state of Queensland, the chief medical officer not only has binding legal authority, but also financial authority over public health matters, and holds a senior position within the state bureaucracy.[26] In Victoria, however, neither of these conditions obtain to the state chief medical officer—it has been argued that the failure to manage hotel quarantine procedures, and in particular the hiring of security personnel instead of public health and medical personnel to oversee the quarantines, was in part because the chief medical officer has no final say in the operation of public health measures in that state.[27]

In light of this, we might consider a few normative requirements for public health leadership as an institutional property. First, leadership roles should comprise a line of coordination for relevant stakeholders, including state authorities pursuing an outbreak response. The primary function of leadership in public health is to promote the nonemergency ends of the institution and, in cases of public health emergency, utilize the tools of the public health state to resolve crises and return a state to public health "peacetime." In this way, the leadership structure of public health should be reflective of its institutional ends. This will depend on the jurisdiction, but following from my argument for the public health state in chapter 5, it is likely that at its highest point leadership for public health will occur on a national level, and serve as a coordinating and executive role between sub-state public health actors (such as provincial, state, and local governments). Public health is local but, as COVID-19 has shown us, the kinds of public health threat that provide a justification for an emergency declaration are likely to span at least nations, if not the world.

Second, leadership must be conferred legitimacy in addition to its legal powers. This provides a positive reason for legislatively authorized, independent offices that act as a coordinating body for public health responses. A chief benefit of a permanent, independent public health office is that it would provide institutional memory over successive outbreaks rather than a series of taskforces and *ad hoc* groups managed in some nations and remove the leadership over public health crises from the partisanship of executive office. In the US, for example, this could be accomplished by relocating and expanding the Office of the Surgeon General and reinvesting that office with appropriate powers to coordinate and make decisions about public health. Alternately, it could be constructed as a new office, with the surgeon general as a member of a leadership council on public health.

Finally, this leadership position must be capable of being held to account in cases of government overreach or error. This stems from the liberty-limiting powers of the public health state, and their capacity to seriously infringe on the rights of individuals. The legal powers of a public health office might be considerable, and so its leadership should be accountable in cases where it oversteps its bounds. Failures of leadership are inevitable, but a key component of rebuilding trust is the ability to hold leaders to account. Ultimately, the institution and its legitimate role are more important than the individuals who occupy leadership positions within that institution, and maintaining trust requires the ability to course correct when the institution goes astray.

This seems an ambitious set of requirements, but in light of the current absence of coordinated leadership, states have an opportunity to develop a more robust and coordinated set of institutions that govern public health. In thinking about war metaphors, war is so important that we relegate the decision-making power to go to war to the highest offices but entrust the operations and conduct of that war to specific and experienced institutional roles. We sorely underappreciate the role of leadership as an element of institutional design in public health. In his tribute to Jonathan Mann, Lawrence Gostin has noted that "leadership and politics" are important elements of public health.[28] Getting the former, however, will require some of the latter.

Conclusions

In the sum of things, wars are fought not with guns and tanks but with people. So too, with public health. A key lesson in pandemics present and past is that public health responses to communicable disease outbreaks may be helped by science but are ultimately responded to and resolved by people. The relationships those people have with those in their care is ultimately more important than any virologist's sample collection or any epidemiologist's model.

In this chapter I argued that an account of just health security establishes two things. The first is that healthcare workers accept, as part of their professional role, some personal liability in aid of resolving a public health emergency. However, that liability is not unlimited, and a public health action and response is unjust insofar as it exceeds that liability.

Second, I maintained that the legitimacy of the state confers a need for adequate leadership over a public health emergency. That leadership should inform institutional design, comprise a line of coordination for the relevant stakeholders in a response, be legislatively authorized and with the appropriate legitimacy. These qualities provide a backbone against which the remainder of an institution rests and generate the norms that individuals believe we have lost in public health. However, given the long absence of real leadership as an institutional quality, it is uncertain when—or if—that loss occurred.

9   Peace in Public Health

The *jus post bellum*, as it is called, is the ethics of ending war.[1] In this penultimate chapter, I continue exploring the relationship between military ethics and public health by asking: if we take this question of war seriously, what should the end of a public health emergency look like?

The importance of this question has important antecedents. In almost all cases, even once the immediate danger has passed, public health emergencies are catastrophes. The 2013–2016 Ebola outbreak devastated the Western African nations of Guinea, Liberia, and Sierra Leone. And the long-term effects of Zika virus in Latin America, which affected neonatal development, will be present for a generation. The rise of "long COVID" will potentially lead to cognitive deficits and organ injury for many millions of people worldwide.

And yet, we appear to be very bad at ending public health crises. Once antiretrovirals were available to a select group of patients, HIV/AIDS stopped being a crisis—for those who made it one publicly. Writing in 2022, Gregg Gonsalves noted of HIV/AIDS that

> the AIDS pandemic didn't fully end. In a way it did end for many white middle-class gay men like us; we had access to these drugs and to good medical care overall and could start to think about getting back to normal. But AIDS still lingered and flourished in America in places that were easy for people like us to ignore.[2]

So too, with COVID-19, have things gone back to normal—for some. In his editorial critiquing the Biden administration's leadership in the pandemic, *Science* editor in chief Holden Thorp claimed the response of the administration

> has been a clumsy pivot to a message that politicians always turn to: personal responsibility. Get vaccinated, get boosted, wear a mask, get a prescription for the antiviral Paxlovid—if you want to. This may be fine if you have a healthy

immune system, great health insurance, and the ability to navigate the US health care system. But what about everyone else?[3]

In both cases, the crisis presented by infectious disease ends because it stops threatening certain powerful kinds of people, and it is left to burn through the poor, marginalized, disabled, and racially subordinated communities. As a work of philosophy, however, my question is less about what counts as the "end" of a crisis, but more about what *should* count.

Just war theory has over time incorporated an account of what our obligations are after war to secure a lasting peace. These change somewhat for us when we think about just health security, in part because while the causative agent of disease is the "enemy," that enemy has no assets or territory to forfeit, can give no account of its actions, and cannot be tried. So, our principles are focused more on the harms that were inflicted during a public health emergency, on rebuilding, and preparing for the next crisis.

In this penultimate chapter I will deal with the ethics of ending a public health emergency. I start with the basics of *jus post bellum*: providing terms to end a war, guidance on peace, political reconstruction, and preventing revenge. I follow this through with their application to public health ethics. I conclude with a comment on global responsibility, and what it might mean to hold states accountable for COVID-19.

Jus post Bellum

The aims of the just war are to secure a just peace. Until recently, this was not codified as an independent set of principles. Those principles, the *jus post bellum*, are a series of criteria originally popularized by Brian Orend.[4] Since then, it has grown into a small but diverse literature covering everything from war's end,[5] to the prosecution of war crimes and genocide,[6] to our obligations to rebuild after war.[7] These perspectives have framed ongoing discussion around the obligations states have at the end of a conflict.

The basic tenets around *jus post bellum* emerge from two considerations. First, war's end cannot be unconditional: it oversteps the bounds of justified war to continue until an aggressor has been eliminated or submitted in such a way that it has no power with which to sue for peace. Second, the mere end to war is not the ultimate aim. Rather an ongoing peace is the proper end of war, and indeed connects the end of war to the just cause that motivated it in the first place. These give us a series of criteria to guide what the end of war should look like.

The first criteria is a just end to war. Even wars justly begun might be unjustly ended. A just war that turns into a campaign of extermination, or of totally conquering a sovereign state, is regarded as an extreme violation of the rights of individuals within that territory well beyond a state's rights to defend itself. The domestic analogy here is that if I subdue my attacker my right to self-defense is fulfilled; if I proceed to beat him near to death, I have overstepped what is my right and battered him without just cause. If I beat him near to death and then kidnap his family or burn down his house, likewise I have exceeded my defensive rights.

The next is that a just peace must ensue. This is a peace in which mutual respect between states is restored, and in which all parties can go on to exert their sovereignty in the future. That just peace must also be a "lasting peace," in which the conditions for a return to war are not present, and a good faith effort is made to continue peace indefinitely. While indefinite or perpetual peace is simply unlikely, a just peace is one in which there is some confidence that war will not ensue just as soon as the formalities of a truce are complete.

The third is reparations and justice for the victims. This includes justice for war crimes by leaders and soldiers, and reparations for property destroyed, lives lost, and other harms incurred during war. While many advocates of *jus post bellum* maintain the idea of a "belligerents rebuild" thesis, in which the warring parties are obligated to rebuild, James Pattison has recently defended a thesis in which the international community rebuilds according to their capacity to do so.[8] In light of the fact that our enemy, properly defined, is a non-agential threat in the form of a communicable disease, this is particularly important: we cannot require a duty of the enemy to rebuild because our enemy isn't the kind of thing that can possess duties. Moreover, if we have adequately prepared for and responded to a crisis, then states will almost certainly have engaged in altruistic actions toward their neighbors through pandemic preparedness and response, and thus may require rebuilding themselves as part of preparing for the next pandemic—requiring a coordinating international response.[9] This key departure will become important toward the end of the chapter.

The Ethics of Ending a Public Health Emergency

The first obvious application of *jus post bellum* to public health emergencies is in the end of the emergency. As a matter of policy, in many cases public health emergencies end after a statutory period unless they are renewed. In others, they may continue indefinitely until the relevant authority deems otherwise. However, from a normative perspective we can begin based on what counts as an emergency. If an emergency is exigent, harmful, and overwhelming, then some emergencies cease when they cease to satisfy these criteria. When an event is no longer exigent, harmful, and overwhelming, it ceases to become an emergency.

This might not be enough, however, due to the nature of our threat and the kind of event an emergency declaration constitutes. Just because all three criteria of threat—magnitude, exigency, and capacity to respond—are required to constitute an emergency does not mean the cessation of one eliminates an emergency. Cessation of exigency, for example, may simply be the acceptance of something as now part of the fabric of day-to-day life even if mortality continues to be extremely high. We are seeing this with COVID—it is far from clear emergency conditions have ended, and ERs continue to operate at capacity, but nonetheless we have returned to normal. As was put by virologist Aris Katzourakis, regarding endemic COVID, "Yes, common colds are endemic. So are Lassa fever, malaria and polio. So was smallpox, until vaccines stamped it out."[10]

Rather, an emergency ceases when it ceases to be both harmful and overwhelming. That is, we should not end an emergency before there is a reasonable belief that the danger will not return the second we let our guard down. Writing in June 2022, Martha Lincoln and Lorenzo Servitje caution regarding the lack of enthusiasm in the US for resolving the pandemic beyond letting the virus spread

> Where many pundits have attempted to normalize COVID-19 or make it seem trivial by comparing it to other causes of death, such as cancer and the flu, this is a misleading way of thinking about death at the level of the national population. The impact of COVID-19 has caused a sea change in patterns of mortality in the United States. Indeed, the outsize share of death now caused by an infectious disease could threaten a reversal of the gains we've made in public health over the last seventy-five years. This concerning trend in mortality is not our only cause for concern: as the CDC recently reported, some 1 in 5 Americans who are infected with COVID-19 will experience long COVID symptoms.
>
> To be sure, the way forward is not simple. But the alternative is unacceptable. Now is not the time to seek the upward threshold for accepting pandemic deaths, nor to recalibrate expectations for public health to the standards of the last century. The "new normal" that we're being asked to settle into is no best-case scenario, but a shocking anachronism—a detour into a less healthy and more dangerous past.[11]

Clearly, simply embracing "normal" when it comes to an ongoing and uncontrolled infectious disease outbreak is not just—it does not satisfy just cause, nor does it lead to a lasting "peace." Note, however, that this does not mean that disease eradication is necessary or the only justification for ending a public health emergency. This is partly because some diseases are, at least given our current capacities, ineradicable in virtue of being zoonoses. We can imagine a point in an Ebola outbreak in which a few cases remain, but they are well managed through local contact tracing conducted by members of a community appointed and authorized in a rights-respecting way as part of a traditional public health state. We may be required here to lift the emergency if there is a reasonable belief that the cases that are left are managed to such an extent that the outbreak will ultimately end. We know it will return, so long as great apes, and certain bat species among other animal reservoirs, remain. But the mere possibility that Ebola will return in a new outbreak is not reason to maintain an emergency state.

This also partly addresses what we might consider the public health analogue to the second consideration in *jus post bellum*, of a lasting peace. COVID-19 is a zoonotic pathogen, and since its emergence in the People's Republic of China it has been found in animals indigenous to other continents, such as white-tailed deer.[12] Yet the presence of COVID-19 in white-tailed deer does not provide a reason to capitulate against elimination in humans. Rather, a lasting peace might be thought of as returning to a state where COVID-19 is rare in humans, though it may arise when humans interact with deer populations.

In the case of public health emergencies, a lasting stability has additional components. The principle of last resort has implicit in it the idea that if fulfilled, public health emergencies will be rare; where they are not, there is cause to believe that the public health state has failed to function in some important way.[13] A lasting peace would arguably involve the repair of whatever systems are identified to have led to the emergence of disease, consistent with other moral considerations. That's why, in the case above, it is not merely that low case counts signify an end to a public health emergency. Rather, it must incorporate a reduction in harm with the rise of capacity to prevent the situation from becoming overwhelming again.

Reconstruction and reparations are perhaps the most direct comparison to war we have in the end of public health emergencies. The former should be managed to bring health systems back into repair, allowing them to serve the community under conditions of the rights-respecting public health state. That is, depleted health systems should be reconstructed, and other elements of the state fractured by the emergency should be renewed.

Reparations should also be considered for individuals who were harmed by the actions of authorities during a public health emergency in cases where the authorities failed to exercise appropriate liability for their actions, and under which existing institutional supports are not sufficient to provide compensation. In some cases, this may involve direct compensation in the form of money, employment, or even property. But in larger outbreaks this may be a collective act that is designed to provide restitution to communities devastated either by the coercive actions of public health or neglect by authorities.

Public health emergencies are, finally, traumatic events, and individuals may be subject to harm or rights violations at the hands of the state. This includes the public, but as the COVID-19 pandemic has demonstrated to us, also includes healthcare workers, who may have shouldered the burden for a pandemic for months or even years without reprieve, and whose trust in their own institution may be damaged. Rebuilding trust in the state arguably involves acknowledging the harm—and, potentially, its necessity—and nonetheless providing the basis for affected individuals to return to their lives. This may include accountability in cases where leaders or officials overstep their mandate, and an accounting of institutional failures that exacerbated a crisis.

COVID-19 and International Accountability

This final question of accountability for an emergency has an international component. Pandemics are transnational events, and here I deal with two possible forms of accountability, rather than reparation. First, from individuals; and second, from states.

In chapter 4 I claimed that by and large, most humans are not accountable for their disease state. But this is quite different from being accountable for a policy, or a practice, that causes a significant increase in cases. There may be cases in which, much like the direction of practices that cause war crimes, certain public health officials may be responsible for acts that have exacerbated the pandemic, and were completed with full knowledge of that. In the last chapter I noted the suppression of information by US CDC officials, and the acts of a president to willingly ignore a pandemic with a view to their own electoral performance. These are the kinds of acts for which individuals not only pose a threat but are culpable for knowingly harming others in a way that merely infected individuals are not. And where there are private individuals who may have exacerbated the pandemic or undermined the response to the detriment of vulnerable individuals,[14] these groups and individuals are institutional role holders, and thus they might be held accountable for their role in the public health state and its mandate.

The legal ramifications of this kind of accountability, I set aside here. Instead, we can examine the positive moral reasons for wanting this kind of accountability. The first is that unlike threats between individuals in infection cases, the threats institutional role holders may possess are persistent, structural, and have far-reaching effects. Resolving them, and holding those individuals accountable, is a kind of self-defense against institutions in which individuals who have caused these harms are, where possible, removed from the ability to cause them again. These institutions may be necessary, and justified, but particular actors within them have used their powers to cause unjustified harms.

There is, second, a trust-building exercise in these kinds of accountability exercises. That is, when an institution—even one with a robust moral purpose such as public health—breaks trust with the citizens who have given up some of their autonomy and resources to fund it, there should be an expectation that it will engage in some kind of accountability process to determine where, and how, this trust was broken. Note that I am not talking about mere failure, though I admit it is hard to distinguish this sometimes from broken trust. Institutions can be overwhelmed because what makes a public health emergency so dire is its overwhelming nature. But sometimes, as in the cases above, institutions act in ways that rightfully earn the mistrust of a community. In those cases, trust must be regained.

Finally, there is an expressive component to accountability. Sometimes a public is outraged, and rightly so, by their treatment. As in chapter 7, one of the reasons for this relates to risk and harm. When a public health enterprise imposes undue risk on individuals, it fails to treat them with respect as persons with rights and interests. An accountability process is thus a way, after a fashion, that individuals can be recognized—as can their personhood that was so infringed upon.

What of nations? This is a harder question, given the anarchical state of our international politics. There is, in principle, a mechanism to hold individuals accountable within a state, but between states is more difficult. However, and with the "belligerents pay" thesis above in mind, I think there are reasons to forgo punishment for states.

The first such reason is moral luck. As I described in chapter 4, the distribution of infectious diseases that have pandemic potential is not equal over the world, or its human population. Zoonotic diseases in particular are concentrated around areas of biodiversity, which coincide with developing nations that have survived the colonial projects of others. And retributive projects around infectious disease on the international level must first wrestle with the issue that some nations are simply in the wrong place at the wrong time. If they are threats, they are nonresponsible threats, in that they cannot move from their location in the global biome, nor may they have the resources to guard against all possible threats. Moreover, that lack of capacity was caused by someone else, often the very powers that might now point the finger in the case of the pandemic.

Second, there are perverse incentives to reporting infectious disease outbreaks if punishments are on the table. Reporting a disease event can be a catastrophe for a nation: it undermines tourism, industry, and other central economic projects of a nation. Allowing even for the possibility of indirect punishment of a nation that reports infectious disease threatens the most critical phase of preventing a public health emergency: early detection. It thus violates the necessity and last resort conditions; iteratively, knowing that punishment is a key feature of the end of pandemics may make it harder to prepare for the next.

This returns us to the positive need for an international solution to the end of pandemics and preparedness for what comes next. I cannot envisage a system in which it would be rational for states to enter into measures, for example, that extracted sanctions for pandemic responsibility. Nations in the regions in which zoonotic diseases emerge, particularly in equatorial zones and high biodiversity zones, are unlikely to agree in principle to these kinds of conditions because they are almost certainly unfairly targets; and developed countries would be unwise to impose them, as the data we need to detect pandemic pathogens ultimately comes from those same countries. They might withhold support in the form of physical samples and data, which would jeopardize all of us. But that is their bargaining power, and from the perspective of the arrangement described in chapter 5—but now international—it is not instrumentally rational for us to want to pursue retributive global health security policies when we could better secure our long-term interests without such measures.

Instead, there must be distinctively more restorative measures between countries. Part of the need between countries is that the capacities to detect and respond to pathogens exist worldwide. At the same time, legally binding measures that prevent punitive measures being taken against these countries during outbreaks is needed to incentivize sharing and cooperation. International law requires more carrots to encourage behavior, as the use of sticks in global health works about as well as it does for punishing individual behavior, and perhaps worse given that individual nations can simply opt out of the contract between them in the absence of an overarching system of governance.

Conclusion

In this chapter I dealt with the ends of pandemics. I discussed how we might think about the just end to a pandemic, reparations, and how we might think about accountability for certain particularly egregious acts in a pandemic.

This concludes the main section of the book, taking us from the concept of health security and its justification, to declaring a state of emergency, to acting in a pandemic in liberty-limiting ways, and finally to the end of a pandemic. Throughout, I've attempted to address different ways of thinking about just health security that are inspired by debates in just war theory. In the next chapter, I turn to practical implications of this view, and how it might turn from philosophy into politics.

10 Whose War? Policy and Public Health Politics

The "war on COVID-19" we wanted was mobilization, resources, common goals, political legitimacy, and bold action. The "war on COVID-19" we got was early and transparently false declarations of victory, large numbers of civilian deaths, political suppression, profiteering, and conspiracy, dwindling into defeat. Despite this, I have advocated for a reading of the war metaphor, the analogy between security and health, in fairly close terms. How might we proceed and develop health security—and a series of practices as individuals, groups, nations, and a global community—so that it achieves a set of just ends?

One possibility, obviously, is to abandon the analogy altogether. That, I hope obviously, is not the purpose of this book. Not only is the idea of health as security embedded in our consciousness but it is also consonant with a series of principles that can guide us to just action. As a rhetorical device, the analogy tends to fail. But interpreted as the beginning of a philosophical inquiry, it can be useful.

The theory I have described in this book, as a theory of health security, is demanding. It is based on a position that is ancient, historically grounded, and supported by contemporary moral reasoning. It is demanding, however, because it does not start from a realist position around security and attempt to salvage justice from within that. Rather, it starts from the position of what a just state ought to look like, and then works back from that. Public health is an issue of individual and collective security, but acting on this requires from us a commitment to justice that envisages a robust, rights-respecting public health state; an impersonal account of disease; and commitment to just, brief, and limited emergency acts in those cases where we are threatened, despite our best efforts, by communicable disease, natural disaster, or biological war.

As a philosophical position, it is my hope that this first entry will prompt discussion—there are additional controversies to be explored, the limits of my account to be tested, and so on. My experience with practitioners in the field is that they are practical to a fault: they will pose the question "so what?" This chapter is a reply to them, and it is about health security itself, and what we might do to bring about a just health security. In philosophical parlance, this is a chapter about a kind of non-ideal theory: how we get from where we are today, to where we ought to be. Though my colleagues in philosophy and my colleagues in health security are more or less disjunctive groups, this conclusion, as a reflection, should be applicable for both.

The Poison of Naive Neutrality

Just health security is morally demanding, but it is deliberately morally thin. I described this in chapter 5. As we have seen over the last two years, health security can be apolitical to the point of cruelty: a form of naive neutrality that sees the instrumental value of staying "in the room"—where those rooms are usually rich or powerful spaces in national capitals—as more important than mobilizing political power and running the risk of being shut out of the discussion, even if only temporarily.

By "naive neutrality," I reference "liberal neutrality," a foundational element of political liberalism: governments ought to maintain an attitude of neutrality toward the many conceptions of the good life that are held by the members of society. Health security as it stands has a form of neutrality, but one that is not truly neutral over the potential range of what constitutes the good life. Rather, it is neutral over the political terrain of the current world—which is, itself, far from neutral about substantive ideals of morality. This makes it risk averse over a range of issues that might be construed as partisan within contemporary politics. There is a reason, for example, why in the US health security's position on medical countermeasures is reflected better in the FDA's Animal Rule that allows emergency use of pharmaceuticals without human testing, than in pharmaceutical benefit access to guarantee essential medicines in the US are free at the point of sale to citizens. It is why the dismantling of *Roe v. Wade*, which will almost certainly result in worse maternal outcomes and a loss of essential healthcare facilities that cater to poor women, has not been taken up by the community. There is, fundamentally, a reason why global health security reform "lessons learned" documents often include the need for improved surveillance networks, but rarely universal access to healthcare. There is a reason why health security usually cares more about terrorists securing Ebola than about the lasting disability that results from infectious disease.

As I outlined in chapter 2, this isn't itself surprising. Health security as a discipline is more firmly associated with national security than it is with public health, despite the increasing number of members in the community with backgrounds in public health. It is more at home with the US Department of Defense, in some ways, than with the Department of Health and Human Services. And even when it is affiliated with the latter, it is almost certainly through the National Institutes of Health, which, according to Stobbe, through the 1960s and 1970s was an accomplice in dismantling the power of the US public health service through the surgeon general;[1] or with the American Medical Association, which has itself been an enemy of public health and long opposed substantive reforms in public health and healthcare access.[2] Health security has a fractured identity not just because it is interdisciplinary, but because its practitioners have wildly divergent priorities.

What it means is that the politics in the field have been largely tailored to supporting the status quo, even when that status quo runs counter to the aim of health security itself—preventing pandemics. This is the kind of neutrality I call naive because it takes the political world as it is, as simply the background truth on which health security rests. But the weight of history means that this neutrality is really a form of conservatism. In the US it is true this conservativism is bipartisan in a sense, but that does not fulfill the demands of liberal neutrality, much less the demands of a just health security. Elsewhere in the world, this pattern is mirrored, and health security largely serves prevailing normative trends in society, rather than interact with and, at times, challenge them.

So, what should the findings of this book entail, given the state of the field? I think that depends on how seriously we take the philosophical commitments of just health security, and how closely we tack to this naive neutrality. In what follows, I present three vignettes, each corresponding to a different view of how practical action according to just health security might evolve.

Health Hawks, War Doves

One possible story we could tell that comes out of this is that just health security is taken up robustly by the health security community, or at least a segment of it. Even if practitioners disagree with the details of my account (such as, for example, the epidemiological details of when and where we should declare a public health emergency), they buy into the central premise: that public health is an issue of national security; that this conception of national security is grounded in a vision of a legitimate state that serves the interests of its citizens; and that it takes those citizens' rights as paramount in setting priorities and pursuing public health goals. What comes next is health security that is hawkish on the status of public health in society, but considerably more pacifistic in terms of its national security aspects. Let's call this "health hawks, war doves."

Such a view of health security would see the protection of human welfare as rooted in the institutions of the state, and that health security is best promoted through diverse avenues. It would take, for example, the idea that labor rights are in fact a health security issue, remarking that paid time-off laws have been demonstrated to prevent the spread of infectious disease, and guaranteeing them with the force of law would design a certain number of stay-at-home days in the event of the need for a public health emergency into the basic structure of our institutions. They would advocate for national policies that ensure—if not basic income—then robust unemployment insurance, noting that the temporary collapse of certain key industries such as tourism is guaranteed in event of a pandemic, because these are industries whose constituent feature is the movement of people. It would view a broad set of measures that increase social distance as grounded in essential functions of the state and seek to establish those arms of the state as part of—to borrow a defense phrase—"preparing the battlespace" against a potential emergency. These features would include the modernization of communications to deal with widespread remote work and telehealth; restructuring of educational services to reduce class sizes and prepare teachers for transitions to and from remote education; alternative working conditions that benefit individuals with disabilities and individuals under quarantine alike; and many more.

Centrally, this kind of health security would start from the perspective of advocating for a robust moral vision of the state that is well financed, well prepared, and coordinated in a way that fits its purpose, rather than merely touting individual policies. In this, it would follow national security, which frequently touts a robust vision of the state geared to responding to external armed threats—doing so is neither unexpected nor undesirable when the continuing stability of the state is on the line. This vision of the public health state would promote the claims, already placed by some of my colleagues but in a full-throated and unified way, that access to affordable healthcare is not just a right: it is pandemic preparedness. Responding to climate change is not simply a matter of preserving our environment: it is pandemic preparedness.

Health security practitioners will obviously disagree over the precise contours of which and by how much these statements are true. But critically, and like their national security cousins who disagree on the relative balance of the branches of the armed forces in securing national security, members of the field of health security would take the *existence* of these institutional changes to be fundamental to securing lasting protection from communicable diseases to be uncontroversial. They would not be divided by these differences; and they would not countenance attempts to divide them on these issues.

Moreover, and like their national security cousins, health security hawks of this kind would understand that this cohesion is a political move that advances a shared goal. They would understand that achieving this vision relies on improved bargaining power, and that comes from a unified front that views its mission as partly political. It will not simply describe what it thinks will be the most acceptable vision of health security to those in power, but it will put together what is truly needed to protect the country and then build the political capital to make that happen.

These revisions would mark a sharp change for a wide segment of health security, and in particular the wealthier and more powerful segment of that community. In some nations such as the US, but increasingly Australia and the United Kingdom as well, it would undoubtedly cast health security at least initially in what elements of the political class describe pejoratively as "political" speech, engaging with issues that are subject to partisan conflict. But the choice to avoid those issues is itself a political decision. Revising that decision will create tension, but tension is often necessary to achieve the aims of justice. Either—to use Moehler's terminology—others interact based on mutual interest in long-term cooperation, or they do not. If they do not, things may escalate, but this is a process that politics at times requires.

Beyond this, advocating for stronger international development of global health infrastructure using this approach will take a view to empowering individual countries to govern their own health affairs, and commit to the principle of last resort (as described in chapter 4) by seeking to change the material conditions of public health determinants in a way that respects human rights. Improving healthcare capabilities, education, transit, and basic welfare around the world under this framework becomes essential to a lasting peace against the causative agents of disease. Along the way, access to the relevant scientific knowledge and capacities for individual nations to rapidly screen and detect pathogens would follow, in addition to reforms in trade law to rapidly share life sciences developments that aid in the deployment of technologies to prevent, and respond to, pandemic pathogens. Unlike in conventional national security, in which international relationships are strained between friends and foes, alliances in health are in principle much easier because, in keeping with the findings of this book, the real threat is the causative agent of disease itself.

This will sound like, in addition to health security, a militant view of health writ large. Indeed, it is. But it is militant in the way of collectivist movements worldwide that seek to promote democratic engagement and utilize the state as the means to improve both individual welfare and national productivity. These movements have a long history, and while the Cold War was unkind to them within the US and elsewhere, their modern instantiations still exist. They need not be strictly socialist movements, though some of them are. But any framework of health security that takes seriously the idea that securitized health must respect individual rights will necessarily take the view that the best way to secure ongoing stability in public health is to radically reform our institutions. And it will not tolerate a view of health security that takes human rights to be secondary, or easily forfeited.

Business as Usual, with a Twist

Say that a reader takes this first, optimistic account to be too much. There are reasons to do so: after all, there are many people with substantive moral views that will find my account of the public health state to be too expansive, even if I have argued that this expansiveness is instrumentally rational. What might be done if one takes the main thrust of my argument, but thinks that rather than push for the broadest account of reform we should continue to remain in some sense neutral over larger social questions?

In this case, a number of easy lifts exist that I think would do considerable work, which have received some attention but not as much as they deserve. The first is the focus on refinancing local government health departments. The COVID-19 outbreak has made clear that the level of staffing and resources in local public health departments has led to a dearth of expertise, energy, and time to deal with a major public health outbreak. It is unlikely that COVID-19 is the minimal amount of stress needed to overwhelm this system; a moderate cluster of another communicable disease is likely to do the same to any single health department and threaten the others. (We may find out, with the emergence of monkeypox in 2022.) Refinancing the health departments of local governments, acting in concert with state organizations, would be an easy first lift. It would also be relatively inexpensive: funding contact tracing and basic IT services to keep records would go a long way to harmonizing public health departments countrywide in nations like the United States. Importantly, in countries like the US, new bills to better prepare for pandemics have not taken this option as central to their asks, though the machinery of government is slow and there is still time for change.[3]

The next would be to invest in scientific research into materials and manufacturing for personal protective equipment, nonpharmaceutical public health interventions, and public health decision-making. These topics have been understudied: to the last of them, Francis Collins, the outgoing director of the National Institutes of Health, in a recent exit interview stated in response to what he might have done differently with his time was to fund more social science research.[4] What COVID-19—and Ebola virus disease, and flu, and Zika—show us is that even the most rapid research into vaccines can be fatally undermined unless suppression measures can be achieved, held, and instituted in the most efficient and least invasive way possible, giving time not just for vaccine discovery but manufacture, distribution, and deployment. The unsung heroes of the current pandemic are the public health researchers conducting careful analysis of the broad and varied social distancing measures applied not only nationally but globally in an attempt to parse their relative effectiveness and cost effectiveness. Adding to this, new materials engineering collaborations to come up with cost effective and reusable masks and gowns, and human factors research to make them easier to don and doff, would provide a basis for masking that reduces the load on the public during crisis points.

The core of these aims is to find the largest bang for the limited bucks we will likely have as this pandemic fades. There is a sense in which this is prudent: crises like this can usher in an appetite for austerity. There is nothing that says this need be the case, and certainly other crises have created the space for broad social changes. But knowing where the most good can be done with the smallest amount of effort is a tactic that may be better suited to elements of health security that are for various reasons more risk averse, or lack the knowledge to organize in a way that generates the kind of popular will needed to make broad changes.

The Breakdown

The final option I wish to entertain is what happens if nothing changes. Already, an interminable number of "lessons" have been learned through COVID-19. But these were lessons that arguably should have been learned during H1N1 2009, or SARS, or the Ebola crises of the 1970s and 1980s, or AIDS. The robust changes suggested in the first vignette are hardly different in kind from the demands of the ACT UP movement, albeit framed through a different lens and with the looming and imminent threat of a major climate disaster. Anyone who has spent time working in health security should be moved to tears by the number of lessons we have should have learned but failed to. So, what then?

One troubling thought is that rather than demonstrate the legitimacy of the public health state, the ultimate lesson here is that the current nation-state is by and large incapable of achieving the kinds of institutional goals required of it to secure its own legitimacy. This is most obvious in the US, where I am writing, but it is also likely true in the United Kingdom, potentially in Australia as cases begin to skyrocket there as well, and in many others. Following Moehler's understanding of long-term cooperation, the state—as it is today—might well be run by and for people who do not meet that important fourth criterion of a commitment to long-term cooperation with others. They will deceive, undermine, and even kill those they cannot control. They will allow disabled and poor people to die for their own convenience. And they will mount campaigns to avoid even the most basic changes to a society to prevent the next pandemic—and will do so even if they claim to be working to prevent just that.

If this is true, then a just health security that does not take as its foundation the legitimacy of the state would be needed. The project I have constructed here still has weight: the last resort principle is still applicable because it is grounded primarily in risk, as would be those on liberty-limiting measures. But the architecture of the public health emergency grounded in state declarations would need to be redesigned. I confess I am someone who still holds out hope for a legitimate state, but conversations with friends who hold the opposite view over this pandemic have, if not convinced me, then made me much more sympathetic to their views.

Health security built on this foundation would look profoundly different from its current architecture, but it is not implausible or unanticipated. Radical movements of the 1960s such as the Black Panther Party were liberatory movements whose work included, among other things, the coordination of community health. While the most common images of the Black Panthers are men with guns, Alondra Nelson reminds us, in her book *Body and Soul*, of the critical role the Panthers played in promoting public health within their community.[5] The revised ten-point party platform first drafted by Huey Newton and Bobby Seale came to include explicit mention of the promotion of black health, and requirements that each chapter of the party include the provision of free health clinics. This combined with the Panthers' health activism to insert themselves into the politics of clinical research, and in particular the inclusion of black health needs into the national research agenda and pushback against medicalized racism through the burgeoning genetics movement.

Bobby Seale, in describing the Panthers' development of their platform, describes the division between "what we want" and "what we believe," and the connection between these things. Health security, I contend, frequently lists the former, but omits the latter. This can make our asks at best idiosyncratic—why ask for better and more testing if no one can afford it—and at worst misleading about what it is that matters. Grounding our asks in values—no member of society should be left outside the protective umbrella of pandemic preparedness—situates our policy proposals in ways that can draw attention to and bring diverse groups to the table. The Panthers, in particular, believed in community self-defense and in mutual aid and care in the form, among other things, of school lunches and community medical clinic programs. We tend to remember the former but forget the latter; a health security founded on those ideals would be different from what we see today but is not beyond the realm of political imagination.

The principles of those movements could still be drawn from the work of this book. What would change is the locus of authority and its basis to form an institution of public health within an autonomous community. I don't have the space here to investigate what that change would mean, but the principles of last resort, and of discrimination as it is defined here, would continue to be vital. This is because communities of this kind would have considerably less power to compel their members and would need to adopt strategies that are strongly rights preserving to maintain themselves. I consider this a benefit of these movements, not a drawback. And if that is what it really takes to protect ourselves against the next pandemic, then so be it.

In communities that have survived COVID-19, this may become an increasingly important move as the dominant message that comes from Washington continues to be "you are on your own." Justin Feldman, in one of the only detailed histories of the Biden COVID-19 response to date, noted that around May 2021, when all adults became eligible for the COVID vaccine, the US response changed.[6] As vaccine rates have increased, even with massive case counts and deaths, other countries have followed suit. I suspect that for the most vulnerable, and including many individuals described in chapter 5, there is a sense in which that legitimacy is already gone. How we utilize our bargaining power to make change is thus an open question.

Future Visions of (Public Health) War and Peace

This book is not about COVID-19, but it is singularly inspired by the emergence of that disease and its global spread. What this book seeks to establish is that determining that health is a security issue is a political act. Far from being an attempt to depoliticize health security or public health, it is in fact the opposite, drawing these fields into a set of normative questions that desperately require answering, and are as fundamental as the nature of the state. I have answered them and suggested that a thoroughgoing reading of the ethics of armed conflict tells us something quite different than we might expect from popular depictions of the way security and war are used as metaphors in public health. The ethics of war teaches us that lasting peace is the goal, and that war is at best a tragedy but usually a crime. A contingent pacifist interpretation of health security establishes that human rights and public health are rarely at odds, and that achieving the latter necessarily requires establishing the former.

This provides a series of visions for the future of public health. It is my hope that this book provides an account people will take seriously and operates in good faith in providing a critique of the dominant analysis of health security to date. What comes after is strongly determined by our political will. In the middle of a crisis, it is often hard to see what that might be once we have the space to do anything but survive. Yet it is crucial that we begin discussing what the world should look like when we have counted up the dead. I do not believe for a moment that the world can, or should, go back to normal. Normal is what got us here. The future demands more of us.

Epilogue: Emergency Innovation

This book provides a basic account of just health security, a framework for public health ethics that is in parts derived from a common basis, and in others is inspired by the methodological strategies adopted by military ethics. In the main, this has focused on the arc of decisions that follow preceding, initiating, acting within, and ending a public health emergency: this mirrors the core of just war theory. But there is more to public health ethics, and more to military ethics, than just that. While an extension of these concepts is reserved for future work, one issue became particularly salient during the COVID-19 pandemic: the development and deployment of novel technologies in the service of pandemic response.

If there's one thing people love, it is new toys. And the promise of new technologies is, for most I have encountered in eight years living and working in the US, a vibrant one. There is acknowledgement of risk, but the potential rewards of technologies—as long as Americans possess them first[1]—are always first in their minds. There's a reason why a number of works in and around health security use the phrase "promise and peril,"[2] and, I think, a reason why promise and peril are ordered the way they are.

In the context of communicable disease, technology can absolutely be an asset. The Salk vaccine for polio, smallpox inoculations, and the development of the polymerase chain reaction method to replicate DNA have all been hugely beneficial in the prevention and detection of disease. While antibiotics face an uncertain future,[3] their presence in medicine over the last century has revolutionized everything from common infections to organ transplants, and even in viral epidemics have staved off secondary bacterial infections that may capitalize on and ultimately be the source of a patient's death.

But not all technologies are penicillin: in fact, almost nothing *but* penicillin is like penicillin. Moreover, the benefits of public health are not strictly works of technology. Technology is wonderful, but its application is neither straightforward nor obvious.[4] Jason Schwartz, a vaccine expert at Yale University, is fond of saying that vaccines don't count; vaccinations count.[5] And vaccinations are ultimately very different from vaccines, so different that health security spends comparatively little time even conceiving of the former as technology.

But technology it is, and the connection between basic science and its ultimate implementation is sharpest when pressed into an emergent context. And nowhere, I think, is the war metaphor more heavily used—with the exception of the "warriors on the front lines," perhaps—in public health than when considering innovation during emergencies. In COVID-19 especially, the strategy of the United States writ large has boiled down to waiting for a sufficient number of vaccines to be discovered, authorized for emergency use, and then manufactured and distributed at a scale large enough to vaccinate the population. Even early reports discussed in chapter 7 were not much more optimistic—measures to increase social distance were only a means to endure until the availability of a vaccine.

Consortiums to produce these innovations took on militaristic names: the Israeli "COVID Moonshot" to design protease inhibitors takes its name from the overtly militaristic space race and was echoed in 2021 by the Bipartisan Commission on Biodefense's "Apollo Program for Biodefense"[6]—a Commission chaired by former senator Joe Lieberman, who killed the public option for the Affordable Care Act[7] that would have almost certainly made responding to COVID-19 easier. The Trump Administration's Operation Warp Speed which, while reminiscent of *Star Trek*, was arguably militarized through the lens of that same administration erecting the US Space Force as a branch of the US DOD. Most obviously, a *Wall Street Journal* article described a group of scientists and venture capitalists coordinated by Tom Cahill as pushing a "Manhattan Project" for COVID-19.[8] This last term was mirrored by a memorandum from Peter Navarro, then in the Trump White House, in 2020 describing a "'Manhattan Project' Vaccine Development."[9]

Despite this rhetoric, the connection between military, much less *wartime* innovation and pandemic innovation is tenuous. The aphorism is that "necessity is the mother of innovation," and what could be of greater necessity than defense of the nation? Examples like radar, the atomic bomb, air power, and codebreaking will come to mind as radical innovations completed inside armed conflict. But military innovation *in war* is not as common as these images evoke; their circumstances are much less straightforward than rhetoric suggests.

Typically, bioethics and technology interact most in the context of (1) the ethical, legal, and social implications of technology, and (2) the ethics of particular research protocols used to conduct clinic research during health emergencies. This is a well-trodden path.[10] Rather, what we should do is—as increasingly happens in military ethics—consider the ethics of the institution of biomedical research as it pertains to pandemics.[11]

In this epilogue, I make inroads into just that. I begin with an examination of the two major submetaphors to describe the connection between military and health innovation: the moonshot, and the Manhattan Project. I then examine the current state of play in biomedicine in the US, and worldwide, in preparing for and responding to health emergencies, and how this features into larger norms around health security. I argue that the current metaphors and models of innovation are not just misleading but misplace priorities in pandemic preparedness in a way that privileges interests and preferences other than the justified aims of the public health state.

I then turn to a separate framing of technology in emergencies I dub the "Kalashnikov approach." This draws from the thinking of the Russian technologist and engineer Mikhael Kalashnikov and the rifle that bears his name. It draws from the features of the Russian experience in World War II—a closer analogue to the "block by block" experience of pandemic response in much of the world—and draws lessons, and warnings, from military innovation. It reprioritizes basic innovation and high returns on investment and access over more complex and risky intra-conflict innovation which, while perhaps sometimes permissible, exists like the rest of health security in a climate of neglect of basic social institutions. I conclude with how this might inform future pandemic response.

Moonshots and Manhattan Projects

The moonshot and the Manhattan Project are often invoked in reference to securitized scientific endeavor. The earliest reflection I can find in relation to contemporary biological science comes from Robert Carlson in 2003, and is comparative: Carlson prefers the Apollo Project, which "took place in the public eye, with failures plainly written in smoke and debris in the sky," to the Manhattan Project, which "took place behind barbed wire and was so secret that very few people within the US government and military knew of its existence."[12] Carlson has called for a similarly broad, open vision, in 2000 writing an "Open-Source Biology Letter" to DARPA (paradoxically, part of the US DOD and infamous for a lack of transparency)[13] urging the funding of a revolution in biological technologies.[14]

In 2005, Senate Majority Leader Bill Frist, at a talk at the Nantucket Anthem, spoke about a "Manhattan Project for the 21st Century."[15] It is likely this was strategic: the year before, Republican lawmakers had introduced and passed the Project Bioshield Act first in the Senate, to amend the Public Health Service Act and allocate funds to improve medical countermeasures against diseases that might be used in biological terrorism. This was repeated in 2007 by Michael Osterholm at the University of Minnesota, who with Nicholas Kelley advocated for a Manhattan Project for a universal influenza vaccine.[16]

Today, the metaphor is obviously still alive and well, between COVID-19 Manhattan Projects and cancer moonshots, to describe great and usually expensive undertakings that purport to develop incredible new "game changing" technologies in different arenas. But this framing misses critical elements of each story, its form, and the norms that guided these projects. To begin with the moonshot, most commentators portray the space race as a singular goal to which the US was committed, almost a harkening back to a golden age of American science. But the project was anything but: it was rife with political tension from a Congress that lacked a consensus vision over the value and goals of space exploration, and a tension between the US DOD and NASA over the role of rocketry and its relation to national defense. The moonshot was complicated, and exceedingly messy. The fluctuations in political will and funding would ultimately lead to events like the Challenger disaster, and a complex legacy that has in it everything from increasingly dangerous externalities such as "space trash" to the increasing privatization and militarization of space.[17]

The Manhattan Project, on the other hand, arguably did not suffer from its secrecy. Rather, it was an experiment in scientific governance guided in part by the US military, but also with the enthusiastic participation of the scientists involved. Part of the formation of this project was to give scientists the room to experiment and direct research in line with a very concrete goal of developing a functioning nuclear weapon. But within that, the teams that formed the Manhattan Project—and especially the iconic Los Alamos site—were quite flexible and free with their design. The paradigm of this was Seth

Neddermeyer, allowed to pursue a seeming pipe dream of an implosion-style device involving plutonium, which required him to invent simultaneous detonators and shock physics in the process.[18] Secrecy was, it turns out, not an essential feature of the Manhattan Project *as a scientific project*, though certain aspects of its design as a project were responses to its secrecy.[19]

More importantly, neither the moonshot nor the Manhattan Project were decisive in solving an acute crisis. The Manhattan Project was arguably a response to an urgent situation, namely the threat of a Nazi nuclear weapon (and Japanese attempt at the same). But it outlived those projects, and moreover the architects of the project knew this and continued the project regardless.[20] It is also highly unlikely that the Manhattan Project ended the war in the Pacific, although it was arguably what led to an *unconditional* surrender. The moonshot existed outside of an armed conflict, and while competitive in nature was not pursued under emergent conditions like those of a conventional war. The Manhattan Project took seven years; the Saturn rocket family, eleven years to come to maturity. Both are also deserving of their criticisms, from Eileen Welsome's exhaustive documentation of the human radiation experiments that outlived the Manhattan Project,[21] to Gill Scott-Heron's *Whitey on the Moon*.[22]

The Risks of Emergency Innovation

With this in mind, technology during pandemics is something of a mixed bag. While there are hundreds of drug and vaccine candidates either authorized for use or under investigation in the ongoing COVID pandemic, persistent ongoing issues remain. The first of these is the approval process, and concerns about how truncated such a process can or ought to be to ensure a reasonable expectation of benefit on a population level, while managing potential risks such as serious adverse events.[23] Some suggested solutions, like human infection challenge trials, may cut down on discovery and approval time, but in the process jeopardize the already fragile relationships of trust between the publics—plural, as the public is not a monolith— and the public health-science-governance arrangement of the state.[24] Still other institutional levers such as the Emergency Use Authorization at the US FDA, reformed in the wake of the 2001 anthrax attacks, are potential avenues for rapid approval of drugs but pose risks both medically and reputationally, to providers and governments.[25]

Antivirals and other treatments are in a similar bag. The controversy and spectacle over hydroxychloroquine, which took up roughly 200 clinical trials over the course of 2020 but showed no benefit, was based on a poor set of assertions by French physicians from the outset.[26] The trial of remdesivir, originally designed to treat Ebola virus disease, was stopped by the NIH despite not showing statistically significant survival benefits for patients, but because it met an alternate endpoint of reducing the number of days in hospital for patients that did survive: a controversial decision about what counts in pandemic research.[27]

A flurry of digital contact tracing applications arose in 2020 in response to pressures to reopen the United States, among other jurisdictions. Some of these showed the potential for promise but unlike pharmaceuticals, the majority of these health applications were not subject to rigorous trial designs relative to other nonpharmaceutical public health interventions. This is a serious problem, and for digital contact tracing as part of the larger "big data" movement in public health. Sean McDonald, in 2016, noted that in bringing digital tools into disasters, groups often underestimate the practical and legal implications of digital systems, from data security to operational coordination in the fairness of algorithms.[28] Big data research has been the subject of considerable ethical analysis and demonstrated a need for robust oversight and trials, but in the context of COVID this was lacking.[29]

All of these have exacerbated the mistrust of public health, of science, and of government. This is not the fault, or at least not exclusively the fault, of science and scientists. But as with the impersonal account of disease, we need not issue blame to acknowledge the way that systems are built can be subject to normative critique. And here, there are serious structural issues.

Norms in Need of Change

A key issue for biomedical research is a lack of coordination and prioritization. This is important from the perspective of health security, which has largely regarded the chaos of the life sciences as a benefit.[30] For both these problems, part is internal to the governance of science; part is in virtue of the broader public health landscape.

The internal mechanics of science are disputed, but one popular account goes like this. Scientists publish papers based on two things: the significance of the finding, and its priority. Less interesting findings—by the norms of the field—are worth less; being first is worth much more than being anything else and depending on who you talk to may be the only position worth having. Much of this in contemporary science is backed up first by modern journal culture, and second by the attention media increasingly pays to science during a public health crisis. In this environment, a number of strategies are possible, but two that are common are "followers" and "mavericks." Followers occupy existing epistemic trends and push them forward, where mavericks go in the opposite direction. It has been argued persuasively that both are useful in some degree to the progress of science.[31]

This makes for a series of important dynamics, however, that can become maladaptive in crises. The first is a potential for bandwagoning. We see this with the rapid pursuit of hydroxychloroquine trials over other alternatives; masses of scientists moving toward a single perceived epistemic highpoint that is important both by the norms of the field and society, and while demonstrated to be false consumed excessive scientific resources and was muddied by dozens of poorly constructed studies.[32] Even attempts to synthesize information through reviews have been further frustrated by a paucity of high-quality data, even among published studies, as groups rushed in to compute and then publish their work.[33] Bandwagoning occurs when the prospect of being interesting vastly outweighs the problem of not being first, and there is a prospect of achieving some level of recognition even as a second or third mover. Here, it no longer is rational to pursue untried methods if the tried method produces a result that will always lead to the satisfaction of scientists' instrumental goals. This is not a slight against scientists, moreover: they may still have some pure epistemic goals but shaped in the moment of crisis by other concerns or undermined by the sheer magnitude of a particular prospect.

The second issue is a lack of correspondence between pre-pandemic and intra-pandemic work. A common thread in the ongoing pandemic is a disjunct between priorities in research during not just the COVID-19 pandemic but across many major sources of potential emerging infectious diseases. The issue that arises is how to ensure funding for major infectious disease threats that incorporates a commitment to basic understanding of the diseases themselves. Coronavirus research, famously, has occurred in boom-and-bust cycles around major outbreaks, but with almost no investment in between, despite the warning of SARS.[34]

The third and final issue is what Jason Schwartz has called the turn to the "biomedical model" of public health. This model privileges medical countermeasures and vaccines as the ultimate solution to infectious disease. While eradication of endemic diseases is certainly only achievable through vaccines, or at least has been, the broader collection of public health interventions have not been biomedical in origin.[35] There has been significant investment in basic virology since 2001 to combat particular pathogens thought to be high risk, but never has such an effort been made to understand, trial, and optimize basic public health.[36]

What results is a series of high-investment, low-return trade-offs in many developed nations. The United States and United Kingdom combined have produced the largest number and some of the most promising vaccine candidates for COVID-19. In the background, their health systems are burning up, running out of supplies, and running out of people. Their public health interventions have failed to contain the viruses but not obviously for reasons beyond their control. Pandemic preparedness has made bad investments, focusing on high technology over logistics, planning, and politics; where technology is concerned, neither blue-sky thinking nor ground-level pragmatic concerns have been addressed. The military analogy here is a department of defense with stealth bombers but no pilots; with bullets but no riflemen.

This coordination problem, moreover, is seen in the ways health security research and practice arranges its recommendations. A common point of inflection with military and health innovation is in the infamous "wargame," a combination of physical, virtual, and table-top exercises designed to test theories and innovations against adversaries. These wargames are produced by both government and non-governmental actors and have been conducted on both bioterror incidents[37] and emerging disease pandemics.[38]

What is peculiar about these is the priorities they place on certain forms of innovation and strategy over others. First, recent wargames have emphasized the need for radical medical countermeasures (MCMs) as their highest or near-highest priority: the "Clade X" game run in 2018 made this its first priority; the 2019 "Event 201," unfortunately timed in November 2019 and simulating a coronavirus outbreak, placed it second. The latter of these, moreover, placed overriding emphasis on so-called public-private partnerships, beginning its recommendations with

The next severe pandemic will not only cause great illness and loss of life but could also trigger major cascading economic and societal consequences that could contribute greatly to global impact and suffering. Efforts to prevent such consequences or respond to them as they unfold will require unprecedented levels of collaboration between governments, international organizations, and the private sector. There have been important efforts to engage the private sector in epidemic and outbreak preparedness at the national or regional level. However, there are major unmet global vulnerabilities and international system challenges posed by pandemics that will require new robust forms of public-private cooperation to address.[39]

What are less discussed in these more recent wargames are measures that have been well established as simple but effective means to reduce the burden of infectious disease—including pandemic disease. That is, healthcare access, widely available personal protective equipment, hospital staffing and financing, urban design, workplace access and decontamination, burials, and more: all issues that have been demonstrated as central to infectious disease elsewhere but are largely ignored by wargames of this kind. Event 201 in their recommendations, for example, recommend access to personal protective equipment, but only for transportation workers as part of their third recommendation to maintain trade in a pandemic.

The most charitable explanation of this phenomenon is that these exercises are often model systems that seek to understand a restricted but important part of the pandemic landscape. Event 201 could be interpreted as primarily an exercise in developing issues around public-private relationships. That is, its lack of attention to structural factors is indeed by design, but in the same way a researcher asks one question but not another. The TOPOFF exercise of 2001, for example, did include more detail on personal protective equipment, for example, so not all these exercises are absent these broader questions.[40]

A less charitable, but I suspect more accurate assessment would be that structural factors are messy, hard to model using means that appeal to scientifically minded researchers, and are unfortunately increasingly partisan ideas in American politics—and, indeed, those of many other nations. Moreover, such an assessment would make the wargame itself less charitable, and thus a more bitter pill to swallow for players who are behind the levers of power. Here, the choice is different: still a choice, but based in particular normative commitments that, over the course of this book, I have outlined as central to contemporary health security.

In either case, the choices are a problem. If the latter, it means that an important tool for policymakers is designed around ends that don't comport with the stated aims of public health—preventing, responding to, and ending pandemics. Rather, they are designed to appeal to a particular view of the world and demonstrate a minimal, politically expedient lift for policymakers. All that is needed is more funding for scientific research; all that is needed is for the private sector to be robust enough to replace the public sector (which we acknowledge is underwhelming, but provide no account of *why*, or how, that might change).

This has an analogy in military wargaming. In 2002, the Millennium Challenge was a comprehensive war game designed to test deployment of US forces in the Middle East and was if not explicitly, then implicitly a planning scenario for an invasion of Iran. The team playing opposite the US forces staged incredible initial victories by using low-tech solutions in an early strike on the US Navy and developing prosaic countermeasures to high technology such as using motorcycle couriers that could not be intercepted by aerial surveillance. The challenge was ultimately reconfigured by its designers to *force* a US win, viewed by the leader of the opposition team as a corruption of its initial intent.[41]

In the same vein, recent wargames have a view of pandemic response that encourages one particular normative view of health security but is vulnerable to the ground realities of an actual health crisis. Coverage of health security wargames has noted that the central thing they all held, seemingly mistakenly, was the US doing better than other nations in its response: a belief that seems false in 2021.[42] This is a clue to the possibility that these wargames are designed not to discover what we should do and why, but to enforce a particular version of "why" through the story they tell.

Even the more charitable view, however, is alarming. Writing in 2019, Ronald Klain, once "Ebola Czar" and now White House Chief of Staff, said of Event 201 and Clade X:

> I have growing doubts about these glitzy role-playing events. They create an illusion of improving preparedness, but do they? What ACTUAL progress has been made since the Clade X exercise? People/institutions should be play acting less, engaging policy makers more.[43]

There's an open question that remains about the plethora of wargames that have emerged: even if they accurately simulate a particular interaction in pandemic preparedness, why choose these elements—and what comes of this? Vaccine development during COVID has indeed been rapid, at least for the first few candidates. But under that lies a lack of personal protective equipment, test kits and reagents, surgical gowns, oxygen, and even nurses.[44] Klain's comment drives at a central problem of the previous chapter: that the issues facing health security might be less about the policies or data available, and more about the norms health security itself embodies. This, I suspect, goes for science and innovation as much as it does everything else.

The Kalashnikov Model for Pandemic Innovation

Manhattan projects and Apollo programs are great, but they are grand challenges for great powers. Infectious disease, as health security practitioners love to tell us, is adept at bringing low entire civilizations. It is a faceless, invisible enemy, and the battle for a country is fought in every home, at every workplace, in every congregate setting, and every care facility.

So why on earth would you choose the Manhattan Project? The Manhattan Project was high science, and while its results were far-reaching, they were not adept at fighting a block-by-block war against an enemy. Nuclear weapons are a terrible weapon to use as a comparator when our moral task occurs on home soil. Likewise, the Apollo program may have spin-off technologies (famously, Velcro and Teflon) that are in every home, but none of those technologies got regular Americans closer to the stars.

At the risk of totally breaking the metaphor of health as security, there is one way to reconcile these visions. The weapon in mind is of a kind that *is*, statistically at least, in every American home: the gun. There are approximately 1.2 guns per American. They are easy to acquire, and easy to use for their intended purpose: taking lives.[45] More people know how to shoot, or could use a gun effectively in America, I suspect, than can don and doff a surgical mask appropriately.

In particular, I have in mind the Avtomat Kalashnikova, better known as the AK-47. As an innovation, the AK-47 is an ingenious but understated piece of hardware, and one of the most influential weapons in history. Its inventor, Mikhail Kalashnikov, described his inspiration in its design as arising during recovery from injuries in World War II. Asked by a fellow patient why the Nazis had automatic weapons, but the Red Army had only one rifle for two or three men, Kalashnikov was inspired to build his own: "I was a soldier, and I created a machine gun for a soldier."[46]

What made the AK-47 a machine gun "for a soldier" is what makes it a perfect analogical device for health security. It is designed, first and foremost, for easy mass production using the technology of the 1940s. Its pieces are machined or even stamped. Its reloading system uses a long-stroke piston which, while trading off against some accuracy, is incredibly reliable even under the worst conditions: sand, snow, mud, and water. Its parts can be riveted together, making them relatively easy to repair in a variety of low-resource conditions.

But its mastery is in its ease of use. The fire selector is located on the right of the rifle as a large lever. It doubles as a dust cover, and when in safe mode the charging handle (which pulls the bolt back into position to fire) cannot be retracted. The fire selector's modes, moreover, are arranged ingeniously: safe is all the way up, semiautomatic is all the way down, with full auto in the middle. This means that in a crisis a soldier is more likely to engage semiautomatic than full, which is safer for the soldier and their compatriots. And its trigger system is easy to use with gloves, or with small hands. It is an ideal exercise in human factors, if horrific in its impact.

The Kalashnikov reflects a design philosophy born of Soviet necessity. It does not necessarily reflect Soviet philosophical materialism; rather, it arrived in response to a war—the Eastern Front—that was catastrophically brutal for Russia. It reflects the insights of designers that fought in poor conditions, block by block, in inclement weather, with little training.

Let's consider some of the most critical needs for citizens, more or less everywhere, even if we assume that governments have the wherewithal and political will to institute justified public health emergency measures. They require respiratory protection of some kind and require it in sufficient quantity—either through replacement or sanitization—for the duration of any activities they do need to complete out of doors, or when dealing with sick family. They require a means to disinfect surfaces and potentially themselves. And they potentially require hand and eye protection. Everyone requires these, and they need to be able to be manufactured at scale, anywhere in the world.

Moreover, they need to be able to use these things easily, and without much training. N95 respirators are no good in a pandemic, it turns out, if they aren't able to be taken on and off by just anyone at any time and work no matter what. Hospital signs will notify patients that gloves may be more dangerous than bare hands because donning and doffing personal protective equipment is not trivially easy. Personal protective equipment is, further, no good to most people if it is uncomfortable, because most people aren't medical professionals. Wearability and training are important. Human factors count, and it might be better to make small trade-offs in overall efficacy under proper use, for a much smaller chance of improper use. Or put another way, better they be pretty good and everyone can use them without thinking, than to be really good but only if you use them in a very particular way.

This technology, I suspect, does not exist yet—though after two years, I vouch for the KF94 mask design made and popularized in the Republic of Korea. Prototyping and testing it would not be easy. It would require a broad set of expertise to design, and a wide range of people to test in a broad range of conditions. But it would be a technology for the kind of war like COVID-19 is, and I suspect all infectious disease pandemics will be. It would be a technology anyone could use to defend themselves, and to support the war effort.

To my knowledge, the effort to make better PPE has largely stalled. And the effort to make *comfortable* PPE has never been high on people's list, at least relative to the priorities of major medical funders. This is fine when you are dealing with highly trained professionals who learn how to work with careful, technical equipment and to endure the distraction and discomfort as they work. It is not sufficient for individuals who, even if they train, will never train enough to use PPE appropriately, every time, at the standard of a healthcare worker.

This is the Kalashnikov approach in a nutshell. It does not apply merely to PPE; rather, it takes an approach where:

1. We ask who the technology needs to be for;
2. We determine under what circumstances it needs to be used;
3. We build the best thing we can that fits the broadest possible set of use cases.

Moreover, we build these technologies with a low manufacturing basis. It is not sufficient, for example, to expect individuals to all have 3D printers to make masks. Masks need to be built in places where there may not be 3D printers available. We may need a number of kinds of masks for different environments.

In war, this is a task for the state. The state may make use of private companies but ultimately, they are the arbiters of the kinds of technology needed for the wars they intend, or foresee, fighting. A "lessons learned" plan for the next pandemic is incomplete if it ignores that high technology is, in virtue of its status, ill-suited for a prolonged siege.

Basic STEM for Complex Times

The need for novel therapies, interventions, materials, and strategies in the face of public health crises is not a new issue. And its connection to national security is also quite old. Writing in 1945, Vannevar Bush—himself part of the Manhattan Project—penned a letter to President Roosevelt called *Science the Endless Frontier*.[47] The letter sets forth a justification for basic science as an essential part of the US's postwar national security strategy. It is, Bush argues in *Endless Frontier*, instrumental to the nation's health, wealth, and security.

One of the lesser recognized problems that Bush foresees, however, is a dual public health crisis many of us are intimately familiar with: mental health and overdose. These are obviously not strictly connected but are related. Writing in the 1940s, Bush foresees a strategic problem if the nation becomes mired in mental health and drug overdose crisis. He articulates a vision of basic research into the causes of mental distress, and how to treat individuals suffering from substance abuse with compassion and care. Bush is writing a national security document, one of the foundational documents of the science-security complex. But within it, he treats a very real public health problem.

Bush's insight, however, brings out one lesson that the Manhattan Project can teach us. Bush articulated a program of basic science, conducted for its own sake, involving broad mandates for scientists to research problems deeply, not over years but decades. This is a broader vision born of the Manhattan Project, in which resources were leveraged to provide groups of scientists with the ability to pursue multiyear projects in a productive environment. The agency that would emerge from his vision is not the National Institutes of Health, but the National Science Foundation. While it would be a mistake to pretend that agency has lived up to Bush's dream, this is hardly its fault.

This science, moreover, should be broad spectrum. COVID has demonstrated that pandemics do not just require the life sciences. They challenge materials and chemical engineers, physicists, anthropologists, economists, implementation scientists, psychologists, communication researchers, ecologists, and others. The flurry of biological and epidemiological research has not been as useful as it might have been in the context of the pandemic, not just because incentives within those disciplines are skewed, but because plenty of other knowledge is needed to handle pandemics. That knowledge, moreover, is probably best developed ahead of time, much as we develop operational and doctrinal knowledge ahead of war. We do not need to wait, in almost all cases, for the crisis to start to begin our research.

Notes

Chapter 1

1. The title of this book uses the phrase "Health Security Justice," and not "Just Health Security," owing to a series of conversations with the marketing team at the MIT Press. In brief, the reason for the title being the former is that from an algorithmic perspective, the weight of Norman Daniels's *Just Health Care* and *Just Health* was thought to be an impediment to people finding my book in an age of Google. The choice of title is supposed to reflect that—in this, I confess I am somewhat of a novice, and I have taken my cue from the good people at my publisher.

2. Derrick Bryson Taylor, "A Timeline of the Coronavirus Pandemic," *New York Times*, March 17, 2021, sec. World, https://www.nytimes.com/article/coronavirus-timeline .html.

3. World Health Organization, "Novel Coronavirus (2019-NCoV) Situation Report—1," January 21, 2020, https://www.who.int/docs/default-source/coronaviruse/situation -reports/20200121-sitrep-1-2019-ncov.pdf?sfvrsn=20a99c10_4. Note the WHO inverts the date in this first report, "2019-nCoV." I largely set aside naming conventions around COVID-19.

4. Jon Cohen and Dennis Normile, "New SARS-like Virus in China Triggers Alarm," *Science* 367, no. 6475 (January 17, 2020): 234–235, https://doi.org/10.1126/science .367.6475.234.

5. World Health Organization, "Novel Coronavirus(2019-NCoV) Situation Report—11," January 31, 2020, https://www.who.int/docs/default-source/coronaviruse/situation -reports/20200131-sitrep-11-ncov.pdf?sfvrsn=de7c0f7_4.

6. World Health Organization, "Statement on the Second Meeting of the International Health Regulations (2005) Emergency Committee Regarding the Outbreak of Novel Coronavirus (2019-NCoV)," accessed November 5, 2021, https://www.who .int/news/item/30-01-2020-statement-on-the-second-meeting-of-the-international -health-regulations-(2005)-emergency-committee-regarding-the-outbreak-of-novel-corona virus-(2019-ncov).

7. Massachusetts Department of Public Health, "Man Returning from Wuhan, China Is First Case of 2019 Novel Coronavirus Confirmed in Massachusetts," February 1, 2020, https://www.mass.gov/news/man-returning-from-wuhan-china-is-first-case-of-2019-novel-coronavirus-confirmed-in.

8. World Health Organization, "Novel Coronavirus (2019-NCoV) Situation Report—12," February 1, 2020, https://www.who.int/docs/default-source/coronaviruse/situation-reports/20200201-sitrep-12-ncov.pdf?sfvrsn=273c5d35_2.

9. Wudan Yan and Anne Babe, "What Should the U.S. Learn from South Korea's Covid-19 Success?," Undark Magazine, October 5, 2020, https://undark.org/2020/10/05/south-korea-covid-19-success/.

10. Yascha Mounk, "The Extraordinary Decisions Facing Italian Doctors," *The Atlantic*, March 11, 2020, https://www.theatlantic.com/ideas/archive/2020/03/who-gets-hospital-bed/607807/.

11. Erin Cunningham and Dalton Bennett, "Coronavirus Burial Pits in Iran so Vast That They're Visible from Space," *Washington Post*, accessed October 8, 2020, https://www.washingtonpost.com/graphics/2020/world/iran-coronavirus-outbreak-graves/.

12. N. Ferguson et al., "Report 9: Impact of Non-Pharmaceutical Interventions (NPIs) to Reduce COVID19 Mortality and Healthcare Demand," Report, *20*, March 16, 2020, https://doi.org/10.25561/77482; Caitlin Rivers et al., "Public Health Principles for a Phased Reopening During COVID-19: Guidance for Governors" (Baltimore, MD: Johns Hopkins Center for Health Security, 2020). The "hammer and dance term" comes from a blog post by Tomas Pueyo. See Tomas Pueyo, "Coronavirus: The Hammer and the Dance," Medium, May 28, 2020, https://medium.com/@tomaspueyo/coronavirus-the-hammer-and-the-dance-be9337092b56.

13. Kevin Escandón, Angela L. Rasmussen, Isaac I. Bogoch, Eleanor J. Murray, Karina Escandón, Saskia V. Popescu, and Jason Kindrachuk, "COVID-19 False Dichotomies and a Comprehensive Review of the Evidence regarding Public Health, COVID-19 Symptomatology, SARS-CoV-2 Transmission, Mask Wearing, and Reinfection," *BMC Infectious Diseases* 21 (2021): 710.

14. Bethiana Palma, "Did President Trump Refer to the Coronavirus as a 'Hoax'?," Snopes.com, accessed November 29, 2020, https://www.snopes.com/fact-check/trump-coronavirus-rally-remark/.

15. Yascha Mounk, "Cancel Everything," *The Atlantic*, March 10, 2020, https://www.theatlantic.com/ideas/archive/2020/03/coronavirus-cancel-everything/607675/.

16. Nicholas G. Evans, Zackary D. Berger, Alexandra L. Phelan, and Ross D. Silverman. "Covid-19, Equity, and Inclusiveness." *BMJ (Clinical Research Ed.)* 373 (June 2021): n1631, https://doi.org/10.1136/bmj.n1631.

17. Dylan Scott, "Flattening the Curve Worked—Until It Didn't," *Vox*, December 31, 2020, https://www.vox.com/22180261/covid-19-coronavirus-social-distancing-lock downs-flatten-the-curve.

18. Jeff Pao, "Wuhan Declares 'State of War' against Virus," *Asia Times*, January 24, 2020, https://asiatimes.com/2020/01/wuhan-declares-state-of-war-against-virus/.

19. Jonathan Cheng in Beijing and Chun Han Wong in Hong Kong, "As Virus Spreads, Isolated Taiwan Risks Being a Loophole in War on Epidemics," *Wall Street Journal*, January 22, 2020, sec. World, https://www.wsj.com/articles/taiwan-virus-case-highlights -chinese-efforts-to-exclude-taipei-from-world-health-organization-11579634031.

20. Caitlin Oprysko and Susannah Luthi, "Trump Labels Himself 'a Wartime President' Combating Coronavirus," POLITICO, accessed July 22, 2020, https://www.politico .com/news/2020/03/18/trump-administration-self-swab-coronavirus-tests-135590.

21. Heather Hollingsworth, "Health Workers on COVID-19 Front Lines Once Saluted as Heroes Now Get Threats," *Boston Globe*, September 29, 2021, https://www .bostonglobe.com/2021/09/29/nation/health-workers-covid-19-front-lines-once -saluted-heroes-now-get-threats/.

22. Aishvarya Kavi, "Virus Surge Brings Calls for Trump to Invoke Defense Production Act," *New York Times*, July 22, 2020, sec. U.S., https://www.nytimes.com/2020 /07/22/us/politics/coronavirus-defense-production-act.html.

23. Meredith Wadman et al., "A Rampage through the Body," *Science* 368, no. 6489 (April 24, 2020): 356–360, https://doi.org/10.1126/science.368.6489.356.

24. Tom Brook, "A Run through the Virus 'Warzone' of New York," *BBC News*, 2020, accessed November 5, 2021, https://www.bbc.com/news/av/world-us-canada -52319184.

25. Jonathan M. Marron, Don S. Dizon, Banu Symington, Michael A. Thompson, and Abby R. Rosenberg, "Waging War on War Metaphors in Cancer and COVID-19," *JCO Oncology Practice*, July 2020, OP.20.00542, https://doi.org/10.1200/OP.20.00542.

26. Matt Bille and Erika Lishock, *The First Space Race: Launching the World's First Satellites* (Lubbock: Texas A&M University Press, 2004), 3–4.

27. W. S. Hotchkiss, "The American Medical Association and the War on AIDS," *Public Health Reports* 103, no. 3 (1988): 282–88; John J. Casey et al., "The War on Severe Acute Respiratory Syndrome: United States Forces Korea's Campaign Plan," *Military Medicine* 171, no. 2 (February 2006): 131–135, https://doi.org/10.7205/milmed.171.2 .131; Marcus E. H. Ong, "War on SARS: A Singapore Experience," *CJEM* 6, no. 1 (January 2004): 31–37, https://doi.org/10.1017/s1481803500008873; Nicholas Greig Evans, "Ebola: From Public Health Crisis to National Security Threat," in *Biological Threats in the 21st Century*, ed. Filippa Lentzos (London: Imperial College Press, 2016), 277–292,

https://doi.org/10.1142/9781783269488_0017; Brigitte Nerlich and Richard James, "'The Post-Antibiotic Apocalypse' and the 'War on Superbugs': Catastrophe Discourse in Microbiology, Its Rhetorical Form and Political Function," *Public Understanding of Science*, November 3, 2008, https://doi.org/10.1177/0963662507087974.

28. Colin McInnes, "The Many Meanings of Health Security," in *Routledge Handbook of Global Health Security*, ed. Simon Rushton and Jeremy Youde (New York: Routledge, 2014), 3–17, https://doi.org/10.4324/9780203078563.ch1.

29. World Health Organization, "WHO Coronavirus (COVID-19) Dashboard," 2022, https://covid19.who.int.

30. Congressional Research Service, "Unemployment Rates during the COVID-19 Pandemic," 2022, https://sgp.fas.org/crs/misc/R46554.pdf.

31. Evans et al., "Covid-19," https://doi.org/10.1136/bmj.n1631.

32. Robin Blades. "An Unexpected Pandemic Side Effect in Peru: A Comeback For TB," *NPR*, April 28, 2021, https://www.npr.org/sections/goatsandsoda/2021/04/28/988742791/an-unexpected-pandemic-side-effect-in-peru-a-comeback-for-tb.

33. Jeffrey Kluger, "Domestic Violence and COVID-19: The Pandemic within the Pandemic," *Time*, accessed January 30, 2022, https://time.com/5928539/domestic-violence-covid-19/.

34. World Bank, "Urgent, Effective Action Required to Quell the Impact of COVID-19 on Education Worldwide," 2022, https://www.worldbank.org/en/news/immersive-story/2021/01/22/urgent-effective-action-required-to-quell-the-impact-of-covid-19-on-education-worldwide.

35. Congressional Research Service, "Unemployment Rates."

36. Congressional Research Service. "Unemployment Rates," 10–14.

37. Matthew L. Bosworth, Daniel Ayoubkhani, Vahé Nafilyan, Josephine Foubert, Myer Glickman, Calum Davey, and Hannah Kuper, "Deaths Involving COVID-19 by Self-Reported Disability Status during the First Two Waves of the COVID-19 Pandemic in England: A Retrospective, Population-Based Cohort Study," *The Lancet Public Health* 6, no. 11 (November 1, 2021): e817–825, https://doi.org/10.1016/S2468-2667(21)00206-1; Ian Sample, "People with Learning Disabilities in England 'Have Eight Times Covid Death Rate,'" *The Guardian*, July 15, 2021, sec. Society, https://www.theguardian.com/society/2021/jul/15/people-with-learning-disabilities-in-england-have-eight-times-covid-death-rate; The Health Foundation, "6 out of 10 People Who Have Died from COVID-19 Are Disabled," February 11, 2021, https://www.health.org.uk/news-and-comment/news/6-out-of-10-people-who-have-died-from-covid-19-are-disabled.

38. Hereth et. al., "Long Covid and Disability: A Brave New World," *BMJ* (forthcoming).

39. Katrina Megget. "How New Zealand's Covid-19 Strategy Failed Māori People," *BMJ* 376 (January 25, 2022): o180, https://doi.org/10.1136/bmj.o180.

40. Anna Rouw, Jennifer Kates, Adam Wexler, and Joshua Michaud, "Tracking Global COVID-19 Vaccine Equity: An Update | KFF," September 22, 2021, https://www.kff.org/coronavirus-covid-19/issue-brief/tracking-global-covid-19-vaccine-equity-an-update/.

41. Olivia Goldhill, "We Have Enough Covid Vaccines for Most of the World, but Rich Countries Are Stockpiling More Than They Need for Boosters," *STAT* (blog), December 13, 2021, https://www.statnews.com/2021/12/13/we-have-enough-covid-vaccines-for-most-of-world-but-rich-countries-stockpiling-more-than-they-need/.

42. Lorna Weir, "A Genealogy of Global Health Security," *International Political Sociology* 6, no. 3 (September 1, 2012): 333.

43. Lorna Weir, "Inventing Global Health Security, 1994–2005," in *Routledge Handbook of Global Health Security*, ed. Simon Rushton and Jeremy Youde (New York: Routledge, 2014), 24–25.

44. WHO, *Health Security*, 2022, https://www.who.int/health-topics/health-security#tab=tab_1.

45. Nicholas Greig Evans and Thomas Inglesby, "Biosecurity and Public Health Ethics Issues Raised by Biological Threats," in *The Oxford Handbook of Public Health Ethics*, ed. Anna C. Mastroianni, Jeffrey P. Kahn, and Nancy E. Kass (Oxford: Oxford University Press, 2019), 773–785, https://doi.org/10.1093/oxfordhb/9780190245191.013.67.

46. There has been a small literature on agro-terrorism, the use of biological weapons on plants and animals. See, e.g., Carl Ungerer and Dallas Rogers, "The Threat of Agroterrorism to Australia: A Preliminary Assessment," *Studies in Conflict & Terrorism* 29, no. 2 (March 2006): 147–163, https://doi.org/10.1080/10576100500497012; Njiruh Nthakanio and Wakhungu Jacob, "Emergence of Bio/Agro-Terrorism in Kenya," *Annual Research & Review in Biology* 15, no. 6 (2017): 1–12, https://doi.org/10.9734/arrb/2017/34167; R. G. Reeves et al., "Agricultural Research, or a New Bioweapon System?," *Science* 362, no. 6410 (October 2018): 35–37, https://doi.org/10.1126/science.aat7664.

47. See, e.g., Jonathan B. Tucker, *Scourge: The Once and Future Threat of Smallpox*, reprint ed. (New York: Grove Press, 2002), 191–193.

48. See, e.g., Nicholas Greig Evans, Marc Lipsitch, and Meira Levinson, "The Ethics of Biosafety Considerations in Gain-of-Function Research Resulting in the Creation of Potential Pandemic Pathogens," *Journal of Medical Ethics* 41, no. 11 (November 2015): 901–908, https://doi.org/10.1136/medethics-2014-102619; Nicholas Greig Evans, "Models of Scientific and Technological Review for the Biological and Toxin Weapons Convention," *The Nonproliferation Review* 26, no. 3–4 (October 2019): 351–366, https://doi.org/10.1080/10736700.2019.1662609; Nicholas Greig Evans,

"Great Expectations—Ethics, Avian Flu and the Value of Progress," *Journal of Medical Ethics* 39, no. 4 (March 2013): 209–213, https://doi.org/10.1136/medethics-2012 -100712; Evans and Inglesby, "Biosecurity," https://doi.org/10.1093/oxfordhb /9780190245191.013.67.

49. "There Are Two Sides to Biodefence," *Nature* 422, no. 6932 (April 2003): 545, https://doi.org/10.1038/422545b.

50. Nicholas G. Evans, "'But Nature Started It': Examining Taubenberger and Morens' View on Influenza A Virus and Dual-Use Research of Concern," *MBio* 4, no. 4 (August 30, 2013), https://doi.org/10.1128/mBio.00547-13.

51. Alejandra Mancilla, "Samuel Pufendorf and the Right of Necessity," *Aporia* 3 (2012): 47–64.

52. John D. Banusiewicz, "Hagel to Address 'Threat Multiplier' of Climate Change," *Defense News*, October 13, 2014, https://www.defense.gov/News/News-Stories/Article /Article/603440/.

53. Sadie J. Ryan et al., "Global Expansion and Redistribution of Aedes-Borne Virus Transmission Risk with Climate Change," *PLOS Neglected Tropical Diseases* 13, no. 3 (March 28, 2019): e0007213, https://doi.org/10.1371/journal.pntd.0007213.

54. Megan Scudellari, "Self-Destructing Mosquitoes and Sterilized Rodents: The Promise of Gene Drives," *Nature* 571, no. 7764 (July 9, 2019): 160–162, https://doi .org/10.1038/d41586-019-02087-5; US Centers for Disease Control and Prevention, "Fighting the World's Deadliest Animal," 2019, https://www.cdc.gov/globalhealth /stories/world-deadliest-animal.html.

55. Larry M. Bush and Maria T. Perez, "The Anthrax Attacks 10 Years Later," *Annals of Internal Medicine* 156, no. 1_Part_1 (January 3, 2012): 41–44, https://doi.org/10.7326 /0003-4819-155-12-201112200-00373; Thomas V. Inglesby et al., "Anthrax as a Biological Weapon, 2002: Updated Recommendations for Management," *JAMA* 287, no. 17 (May 1, 2002): 2236, https://doi.org/10.1001/jama.287.17.2236; Thomas V. Inglesby et al., "Anthrax as a Biological Weapon: Medical and Public Health Management," *JAMA* 281, no. 18 (May 12, 1999): 1735, https://doi.org/10.1001/jama.281.18.1735.

56. Evans and Inglesby, "Biosecurity"; Amy L. Fairchild and Ronald Bayer, "Ethics and the Conduct of Public Health Surveillance," *Science* 303, no. 5658 (January 2004): 631–632, https://doi.org/10.1126/science.1094038; George J. Annas, *Worst Case Bioethics: Death, Disaster, and Public Health* (New York: Oxford University Press, 2010); James F. Childress et al., "Public Health Ethics: Mapping the Terrain," *Journal of Law, Medicine & Ethics* 30, no. 2 (June 2002): 170–178, https://doi.org/10.1111 /j.1748-720X.2002.tb00384.x; Nancy E. Kass, "Public Health Ethics From Foundations and Frameworks to Justice and Global Public Health," *Journal of Law, Medicine & Ethics* 32, no. 2 (June 2004): 232–242, https://doi.org/10.1111/j.1748-720X.2004 .tb00470.x; Lawrence Gostin, "Public Health Strategies for Pandemic Influenza:

Ethics and the Law," *JAMA* 295, no. 14 (April 12, 2006): 1700–1704, https://doi.org/10.1001/jama.295.14.1700; Matthew K. Wynia, "Ethics and Public Health Emergencies: Restrictions on Liberty," *American Journal of Bioethics: AJOB* 7, no. 2 (February 2007): 1–5, https://doi.org/10.1080/15265160701577603; James G. Hodge, "Bioterrorism Law and Policy: Critical Choices in Public Health," *Journal of Law, Medicine & Ethics* 30, no. 2 (2002): 254–261, https://doi.org/10.1111/j.1748-720X.2002.tb00391.x; Lawrence O. Gostin and Madison Powers, "What Does Social Justice Require for the Public's Health? Public Health Ethics and Policy Imperatives," *Health Affairs* 25, no. 4 (July 1, 2006): 1053–1060, https://doi.org/10.1377/hlthaff.25.4.1053.

57. Childress et al., "Public Health Ethics."

58. Lawrence O. Gostin, "The Model State Emergency Health Powers Act: Public Health and Civil Liberties in a Time of Terrorism," *Health Matrix*, 2003, http://heinonline.org/hol-cgi-bin/get_pdf.cgi?handle=hein.journals/hmax13&section=7; Lawrence O. Gostin et al., "The Model State Emergency Health Powers Act: Planning for and Response to Bioterrorism and Naturally Occurring Infectious Diseases," *JAMA* 288, no. 5 (August 7, 2002): 622–628, https://doi.org/10.1001/jama.288.5.622.

Chapter 2

1. Jamaji C. Nwanaji-Enwerem, Joseph G. Allen, and Paloma I. Beamer, "Another Invisible Enemy Indoors: COVID-19, Human Health, the Home, and United States Indoor Air Policy," *Journal of Exposure Science & Environmental Epidemiology* 30, no. 5 (September 2020): 773–775, https://doi.org/10.1038/s41370-020-0247-x.

2. "Meet the Heroes of the Front Lines," *Time*, 2020, https://time.com/collection/coronavirus-heroes/.

3. James J. Kimble, "Perspective | The Real Lesson of World War II for Mobilizing against Covid-19," *Washington Post*, accessed October 19, 2020, https://www.washingtonpost.com/outlook/2020/03/25/real-lesson-world-war-ii-mobilizing-against-covid-19/.

4. Rob Copeland, "The Secret Group of Scientists and Billionaires Pushing a Manhattan Project for Covid-19—WSJ," *Wall Street Journal*, April 27, 2020, https://www.wsj.com/articles/the-secret-group-of-scientists-and-billionaires-pushing-trump-on-a-covid-19-plan-11587998993.

5. National Institutes of Health, "NIH Director: Defeating COVID-19 Requires Unprecedented Action and Collaboration," National Institutes of Health (NIH), May 18, 2020, https://www.nih.gov/news-events/news-releases/nih-director-defeating-covid-19-requires-unprecedented-action-collaboration.

6. Tom Frieden, "Dr. Tom Frieden: There's a Long War Ahead and Our Covid-19 Response Must Adapt—CNN," March 22, 2020, https://www.cnn.com/2020/03/20/health/coronavirus-response-must-adapt-frieden-analysis/index.html.

7. Jennifer Khan, "The New York Times," *New York Times*, April 20, 2020, sec. Magazine, https://www.nytimes.com/interactive/2020/uri/embeddedinteractive/a62994db
-13b3-5786-8951-607b6550399b?.

8. Rita Floyd, *The Morality of Security: A Theory of Just Securitization* (Cambridge: Cambridge University Press, 2019).

9. This is related to what effective altruists in health security might call tractability but is not the same: it is less about whether securitization is an effective means to achieve some goal, so much as what its effects are, intended or not. See, e.g., William MacAskill, *Doing Good Better: How Effective Altruism Can Help You Help Others, Do Work That Matters, and Make Smarter Choices about Giving Back* (New York: Norton, 2015).

10. Ian Loader and Neil Walker, *Civilizing Security* (Cambridge: Cambridge University Press, 2007), 10–12.

11. Barry Buzan, Ole Wæver, and Jaap De Wilde, *Security: A New Framework for Analysis*, UK ed. (Boulder, CO: Lynne Rienner Publishers, 1997), 5. See Christian Enemark, *Biosecurity Dilemmas: Dreaded Diseases, Ethical Responses, and the Health of Nations*, illus. ed. (Washington, DC: Georgetown University Press, 2017), 98.

12. The role of speech acts in securitization is also represented by Balzaq, who defines it as a process by which

> an articulated assemblage of practices whereby heuristic artefacts (metaphors, policy tools, image repertoires, analogies, stereotypes, emotions, etc.) are contextually mobilised by a securitizing actor, who works to prompt an audience to build a coherent network of implications (feelings, sensations, thoughts, and intuitions) about the critical vulnerability of a referent object, that concurs with the securitizing actor's reasons for choices and actions, by investing the referent subject with such an aura of unprecedented threatening complexion that a customised policy must be immediately undertaken to block it.

See Thierry Balzacq, ed., *Securitization Theory: How Security Problems Emerge and Dissolve* (London: Routledge, 2010), 3.

13. Cf. Michael J. Selgelid and Christian Enemark, "Infectious Diseases, Security and Ethics: The Case of Hiv/Aids," *Bioethics* 22, no. 9 (November 2008): 457–465, https://doi.org/10.1111/j.1467-8519.2008.00696.x.

14. J. L. Austin, *How to Do Things with Words: Second Edition*, ed. J. O. Urmson and Marina Sbisà (Cambridge, MA: Harvard University Press, 1975).

15. This construction from Rae Langton, "Beyond Belief: Pragmatics in Hate Speech and Pornography," in *Speech and Harm: Controversies Over Free Speech*, ed. Mary Kate McGowan and Ishani Maitra (Oxford: Oxford University Press, 2012), 72–93, 75.

16. In the positive domain, see, e.g., Ian Loader and Neil Walker, *Civilizing Security* (Cambridge: Cambridge University Press, 2007). Simon Rushton's recent book is not necessarily *positive* about the prospects of health security, but he does not consider it viable to abandon it wholesale, and thus attempts to find what might be useful about

securitizing health. Simon Rushton, *Security and Public Health* (Cambridge, MA: Polity, 2019).

17. See, e.g., Colin McInnes, "The Many Meanings of Health Security," in *Routledge Handbook of Global Health Security*, ed. Simon Rushton and Jeremy Youde (New York: Routledge, 2014), 11.

18. Lorna Weir, "A Genealogy of Global Health Security," *International Political Sociology* 6, no. 3 (September 1, 2012), 333.

19. Lorna Weir, "Inventing Global Health Security, 1994–2005," in *Routledge Handbook of Global Health Security*, ed. Simon Rushton and Jeremy Youde (New York: Routledge, 2014), 24–25.

20. Colin McInnes and Kelley Lee, "Health, Security and Foreign Policy," *Review of International Studies* 32, no. 1 (January 2006): 5–23.

21. Argentina et al., "Considerations and Points of Consensus between Argentina, Bolivia, Brazil, Chile, Colombia, Ecuador, Paraguay, Peru, Uruguay, and Venezuela with Regard to Document A/IHR/IGWG/2/2, of 24 January 2005 (Review and Approval of Proposed Amendments to the IHR—Proposal by the Chair" (Geneva, Switzerland: World Health Assembly, January 2005), https://www.who.int/ihr/revisionprocess/en glishmontevideo.pdf.

22. Argentina et al., "Considerations and Points of Consensus," 1.

23. Amanda Moodie and Nima Gerami, *Rethinking Health Security after COVID-19* (Oxford: Blavatnik School of Government, 2021).

24. Christian Enemark, "Ebola, Disease-Control, and the Security Council: From Securitization to Securing Circulation," *Journal of Global Security Studies* 2, no. 2 (April 1, 2017): 137–149, https://doi.org/10.1093/jogss/ogw030; Sarathi Kalra et al., "The Emergence of Ebola as a Global Health Security Threat: From 'Lessons Learned' to Coordinated Multilateral Containment Efforts," *Journal of Global Infectious Diseases* 6, no. 4 (2014): 164–177, https://doi.org/10.4103/0974-777X.145247; Anne Roemer-Mahler and Stefan Elbe, "The Race for Ebola Drugs: Pharmaceuticals, Security and Global Health Governance," *Third World Quarterly* 37, no. 3 (March 3, 2016): 487–506, https://doi .org/10.1080/01436597.2015.1111136.

25. Efthimios Parasidis, "Public Health Law and Institutional Vaccine Skepticism," *Journal of Health Politics, Policy and Law* 41, no. 6 (December 1, 2016): 1137–1149, https://doi.org/10.1215/03616878-3666204.

26. Nicholas G. Evans, Kelly Hills, and Adam C. Levine, "How Should the WHO Guide Access and Benefit Sharing During Infectious Disease Outbreaks?," *AMA Journal of Ethics* 22, no. 1 (January 1, 2020): 28–35, https://doi.org/10.1001/amajethics.2020.28.

27. Moodie and Germai, *Rethinking Health Security*, 12–14.

28. Scott Burris and Edwin Cameron, "The Case Against Criminalization of HIV Transmission," *JAMA* 300, no. 5 (August 6, 2008): 578–581, https://doi.org/10.1001 /jama.300.5.578.

29. Leo Beletsky and Corey S. Davis, "Today's Fentanyl Crisis: Prohibition's Iron Law, Revisited—PubMed—NCBI," *International Journal of Drug Policy* 46 (August 2017): 156–159.

30. Weir, "Inventing Global Health Security," 24. See also Alexander Kelle, "Securitization of International Public Health: Implications for Global Health Governance and the Biological Weapons Prohibition Regime," *Global Governance* 13, no. 2 (2007): 217–235.

31. Weir, "Inventing Global Health Security," 24–25.

32. Sally Haslanger, "What Good Are Our Intuitions?," *Aristotelian Society Supplementary Volume* 80, no. 1 (2006): 95. See also Sally Haslanger, *Resisting Reality: Social Construction and Social Critique* (Oxford: Oxford University Press, 2012), https://doi .org/10.1093/acprof:oso/9780199892631.001.0001.

33. Susan Sontag, *Illness as Metaphor and AIDS and Its Metaphors* (New York: Farrar, Straus and Giroux, 2013), 10.

34. Ken Dilanian, "U.S. Intel Agencies Warned of Rising Risk of Outbreak like Coronavirus," NBC News, February 28, 2020, https://www.nbcnews.com/politics/national -security/u-s-intel-agencies-warned-rising-risk-outbreak-coronavirus-n1144891; Tal Axelrod, "Intel Reports Going Back to January Warned of Coronavirus Threat | TheHill," The Hill, March 20, 2020, https://thehill.com/policy/healthcare/488763-intel -reports-going-back-to-january-warned-of-coronavirus-threat.

35. Clive Seale, "Sporting Cancer: Struggle Language in News Reports of People with Cancer," *Sociology of Health & Illness* 23, no. 3 (2001): 308–329. There is also a parallel literature on medical metaphors used around survivors of physical violence, including in armed conflict. See, e.g., Karmen Erjavec and Zala Volčič, "'Target', 'Cancer' and 'Warrior': Exploring Painful Metaphors of Self-Presentation Used by Girls Born of War Rape," *Discourse & Society* 21, no. 5 (September 1, 2010): 524–543, https://doi.org/10 .1177/0957926510373981.

36. Ed Yong, "Immunology Is Where Intuition Goes to Die," *The Atlantic*, August 5, 2020, https://www.theatlantic.com/health/archive/2020/08/covid-19-immunity-is-the -pandemics-central-mystery/614956/.

37. Caitlin Oprysko and Susannah Luthi, "Trump Labels Himself 'A Wartime President' Combating Coronavirus," POLITICO, accessed July 22, 2020, https://www.politico.com /news/2020/03/18/trump-administration-self-swab-coronavirus-tests-135590.

38. James Hohmann, "British, Canadian and U.S. Leaders Cite World War II to Make Very Different Points about Coronavirus," *Washington Post*, accessed August 5, 2020,

https://www.washingtonpost.com/news/powerpost/paloma/daily-202/2020/04/06
/daily-202-british-canadian-and-u-s-leaders-cite-world-war-ii-to-make-very-different
-points-about-coronavirus/5e8abef088e0fa101a75b5a8/.

39. Gregory D. Koblentz and Michael Hunzeker, "National Security in the Age of Pandemics," Defense One, accessed July 28, 2020, https://www.defenseone.com/ideas/2020/04/national-security-age-pandemics/164365/.

40. Washington, *Medical Apartheid*; Mike Stobbe, *Surgeon General's Warning: How Politics Crippled the Nation's Doctor* (Oakland: University of California Press, 2014).

41. Walzer, *Just and Unjust Wars*, 22.

42. Laura Spinney, *Pale Rider: The Spanish Flu of 1918 and How It Changed the World* (New York: PublicAffairs, 2017), 77.

43. Jeffery K. Taubenberger and David M. Morens, "1918 Influenza: The Mother of All Pandemics," *Emerging Infectious Diseases* 12, no. 1 (January 2006): 15–22, https://doi.org/10.3201/eid1209.050979.

44. Donald R. Hopkins, *Princes and Peasants: Smallpox in History* (Chicago: University of Chicago Press, 1983).

45. US Centers for Disease Control and Prevention, "Burden of Influenza," Centers for Disease Control and Prevention, April 17, 2020, https://www.cdc.gov/flu/about/burden/index.html.

46. Shad Thielman, "Death by Numbers: How Vietnam War and Coronavirus Changed the Way We Mourn," The Conversation, May 15, 2020, http://theconversation.com/death-by-numbers-how-vietnam-war-and-coronavirus-changed-the-way-we-mourn-137675.

47. Martin A. Makary and Michael Daniel, "Medical Error—The Third Leading Cause of Death in the US," *BMJ* 353 (May 3, 2016): i2139, https://doi.org/10.1136/bmj.i2139.

48. Jonathan Herington, "The Concept of Security," in *Ethics and Security Aspects of Infectious Disease Control*, ed. Christian Enemark and Michael J. Selgelid (London: Ashgate, 2012), 7–26.

49. See Jeremy Youde, *Global Health Governance* (Malden, MA: Polity, 2012), 138–140.

50. Giuliana Viglione, "Tens of Thousands of Scientists Are Redeploying to Fight Coronavirus," *Nature News*, March 27, 2020, https://www.nature.com/articles/d41586-020-00905-9.

51. James Hamblin, "The Curve Is Not Flat Enough," *The Atlantic*, March 28, 2020, https://www.theatlantic.com/health/archive/2020/03/coronavirus-forcing-american-hospitals-ration-care/609004/.

52. Nolan D. McCaskill and Miranda Ollstein, "Trump Administration Tells States to Step Up as Governors Plead for Aid," *Politico*, April 5, 2020, https://www.politico.com/news/2020/04/05/white-house-trump-funding-states-coronavirus-165783.

53. Center for Strategic and International Studies,"A Covid-19 Response Corps Can Help Stop the Pandemic," 2020, https://www.csis.org/analysis/covid-19-response-corps-can-help-stop-pandemic.

54. CDC, "Communities, Schools, Workplaces, & Events," Centers for Disease Control and Prevention, April 30, 2020, https://www.cdc.gov/coronavirus/2019-ncov/php/open-america/staffing.html.

55. Boston University, "Epidemiology COVID-19 Response Corps," 2020, https://sites.bu.edu/covid-corps/.

56. NC Government, "NC Gov. Cooper: NC College Students Help Local Governments, Nonprofits with COVID-19 Response," July 9, 2020, https://governor.nc.gov/news/nc-college-students-help-local-governments-nonprofits-covid-19-response.

57. Used here in the economic sense; i.e., an actor that seeks to maximize its profits.

58. Susie Cagle, "How Hospital Monopolies Broke the Health Care System," December 2, 2020, https://www.thenation.com/article/society/coronavirus-health care-consolidation/.

59. P. W. Singer, *Corporate Warriors: The Rise of the Privatized Military Industry*, 2nd ed. (Ithaca, NY: Cornell University Press, 2011).

60. Ned Dobos, *Ethics, Security, and The War-Machine: The True Cost of the Military* (Oxford: Oxford University Press, 2020).

61. Aishvarya Kavi, "Virus Surge Brings Calls for Trump to Invoke Defense Production Act," *New York Times*, July 22, 2020, sec. U.S., https://www.nytimes.com/2020/07/22/us/politics/coronavirus-defense-production-act.html.

62. "The Defense Production Act and the Failure to Prepare for Catastrophic Incidents," *War on the Rocks*, April 14, 2020, https://warontherocks.com/2020/04/the-defense-production-act-and-the-failure-to-prepare-for-catastrophic-incidents/.

63. Ben Finley, "Obama's Executive Orders," *FactCheck.Org* (blog), September 25, 2012, https://www.factcheck.org/2012/09/obamas-executive-orders/.

64. Jim Powell, "Obama's Plan to Seize Control of Our Economy and Our Lives," *Forbes*, accessed August 20, 2020, https://www.forbes.com/sites/jimpowell/2012/04/29/obamas-plan-to-seize-control-of-our-economy-and-our-lives/.

65. RT, "Alex Jones: Obama's Executive Order Facilitates Martial Law," *InfoWars* (blog), March 21, 2012, https://www.infowars.com/alex-jones-obamas-executive-order

-facilitates-martial-law/. The conversation about EO 13603 from the Obama administration, the subject of the controversy, is found at the end of the third hour of the March 21, 2012, show of Alex Jones in his interview with Jerome Corsi, another conspiracy theorist most famous for being "Person 1" in the trial of Roger Stone in 2018.

66. Though as Dobos notes, "imagine" here does a surprising amount of work. See Ned Dobos, *Ethics, Security, and The War-Machine: The True Cost of the Military* (Oxford: Oxford University Press, 2020).

67. "Dr. Tom Frieden: There's a Long War Ahead and Our Covid-19 Response Must Adapt—CNN," accessed July 22, 2020, https://www.cnn.com/2020/03/20/health /coronavirus-response-must-adapt-frieden-analysis/index.html.

68. "Prepare Now for the Long War Against Covid-19," *Bloomberg.com*, March 20, 2020, https://www.bloomberg.com/opinion/articles/2020-03-20/prepare-now-for-the -long-war-against-coronavirus.

69. Micah Zenko, "The Coronavirus Is the Worst Intelligence Failure in U.S. History," *Foreign Policy*, March 25, 2020, https://foreignpolicy.com/2020/03/25/coronavirus-worst -intelligence-failure-us-history-covid-19/.

70. There is a long history of discussion of strategic surprise, arguably tracing back (in the Western canon) to Clauswitz. See Michael I. Handel, "Intelligence and the Problem of Strategic Surprise," *Journal of Strategic Studies* 7, no. 3 (September 1, 1984): 229–281, https://doi.org/10.1080/01402398408437190. In contemporary work, the term can be used quite broadly to describe everything from novel advances in technology to overconfidence against asymmetrically weaker powers such as the Iraqi insurgency starting in 2003. See Phil Williams, "Strategic Surprise and Lessons for Future Contingencies," *Prism* 1, no. 2 (2010): 47068; DOD Defense Science Board, "DSB Summer Study Report on Strategic Surprise" (Office of the Undersecretary of Defense for Acquisition, Technology, and Logistics, July 2015).

71. Seth Lazar, *Sparing Civilians* (Oxford: Oxford University Press, 2016).

72. Walzer, 152–153. See also 128–133 for his analysis of Sidgwick's argument for utility and proportionality, which becomes important later.

73. Nicholas G. Evans, "Covid-19: The Ethics of Clinical Research in Quarantine," *BMJ* 369 (May 29, 2020), https://doi.org/10.1136/bmj.m2060.

74. Kelly Hills, "Rejecting Quarantine," in *Ebola's Message*, ed. Nicholas Greig Evans, Tara C. Smith, and Maimuna S. Majumder (Cambridge, MA: MIT Press, 2016), 217–231.

75. Hamblin, "The Curve Is Not Flat Enough."

76. Yascha Mounk, "The Extraordinary Decisions Facing Italian Doctors," *The Atlantic*, March 11, 2020, https://www.theatlantic.com/ideas/archive/2020/03/who-gets -hospital-bed/607807/.

77. Nicholas Greig Evans and Thomas Inglesby, "Biosecurity and Public Health Ethics Issues Raised by Biological Threats," in *The Oxford Handbook of Public Health Ethics*, ed. Anna C. Mastroianni, Jeffrey P. Kahn, and Nancy E. Kass (Oxford: Oxford University Press, 2019), 773–785, https://doi.org/10.1093/oxfordhb/9780190245191.013.67.

78. Nicholas Rescher, "The Allocation of Exotic Medical Lifesaving Therapy," *Ethics* 79, no. 3 (1969): 173–186.

79. Albert R Jonsen, "The God Squad and the Origins of Transplantation Ethics and Policy," *Journal of Law, Medicine & Ethics* 35, no. 2 (June 2007): 238–240, https://doi .org/10.1111/j.1748-720X.2007.00131.x.

80. Nicholas Greig Evans and Mohamed A. Sekkarie, "Allocating Scarce Medical Resources during Armed Conflict: Ethical Issues," *Disaster and Military Medicine* 3, no. 1 (2017): 5, https://doi.org/10.1186/s40696-017-0033-z; Majd Isreb et al., "Effect of Besiegement on Non-Communicable Diseases: Haemodialysis," *The Lancet* 388, no. 10058 (November 2016): 2350.

81. E. M. M. Bernthal, R. J. Russell, and H. J. A. Draper, "A Qualitative Study of the Use of the Four Quadrant Approach to Assist Ethical Decision-Making during Deployment," *Journal of the Royal Army Medical Corps* 160, no. 2 (2014): 196–202, https://doi .org/10.1136/jramc-2013-000214; Evans and Sekkarie, "Allocating Scarce Medical Resources," *Disaster and Military Medicine* 3, no. 1 (2017): 5, https://doi.org/10.1186 /s40696-017-0033-z; Steven P. Cohen et al., "Diagnoses and Factors Associated with Medical Evacuation and Return to Duty for Service Members Participating in Operation Iraqi Freedom or Operation Enduring Freedom: A Prospective Cohort Study," *The Lancet* 375, no. 9711 (January 2010): 301–309, https://doi.org/10.1016/S0140 -6736(09)61797-9; Christiane Rochon, "Dilemmas in Military Medical Ethics: A Call for Conceptual Clarity," December 2015, https://papyrus.bib.umontreal.ca/xmlui/handle /1866/12795.

82. Floyd, *The Morality of Security*.

Chapter 3

1. Shirley Sze et al., "Ethnicity and Clinical Outcomes in COVID-19: A Systematic Review and Meta-Analysis," *EClinicalMedicine* 0, no. 0 (November 12, 2020), https:// doi.org/10.1016/j.eclinm.2020.100630.

2. Gene Falk et al., "Unemployment Rates During the COVID-19 Pandemic: In Brief" (Washington, DC: Congressional Research Service, 2020); US Bureau of Labor Statistics, "The Employment Situation—November 2020" (Washington, DC: Department of Labor, December 4, 2020).

3. Mark É. Czeisler, "Delay or Avoidance of Medical Care because of COVID-19– Related Concerns—United States, June 2020," *MMWR: Morbidity and Mortality Weekly*

Report 69 (2020), https://doi.org/10.15585/mmwr.mm6936a4; Lisa Rosenbaum, "The Untold Toll—The Pandemic's Effects on Patients without Covid-19," *New England Journal of Medicine* 382, no. 24 (June 11, 2020): 2368–2371, https://doi.org/10.1056/NEJMms2009984.

4. Jennifer Clapp and William G. Moseley, "This Food Crisis Is Different: COVID-19 and the Fragility of the Neoliberal Food Security Order," *Journal of Peasant Studies* 47, no. 7 (November 9, 2020): 1393–1417, https://doi.org/10.1080/03066150.2020.1823838.

5. Bridget Balch, "54 Million People in America Face Food Insecurity during the Pandemic: It Could Have Dire Consequences for Their Health," AAMC, accessed December 15, 2020, https://www.aamc.org/news-insights/54-million-people-america-face-food-insecurity-during-pandemic-it-could-have-dire-consequences-their.

6. Brad Boserup, Mark McKenney, and Adel Elkbuli, "Alarming Trends in US Domestic Violence during the COVID-19 Pandemic," *American Journal of Emergency Medicine* 38, no. 12 (December 1, 2020): 2753–2755, https://doi.org/10.1016/j.ajem.2020.04.077; Yasmin B. Kofman and Dana Rose Garfin, "Home Is Not Always a Haven: The Domestic Violence Crisis amid the COVID-19 Pandemic," *Psychological Trauma: Theory, Research, Practice, and Policy* 12, no. S1 (20200601): S199, https://doi.org/10.1037/tra0000866; Hayley Boxall, Anthony Morgan, and Rick Brown, "The Prevalence of Domestic Violence among Women during the COVID-19 Pandemic," *Australasian Policing* 12, no. 3 (September 2020): 38.

7. UNICEF, *Preventing a Lost Decade: Urgent Action to Reverse the Devastating Impact of COVID-19 on Children and Young People* (Geneva: United Nations, 2021).

8. Melody Schreiber, "'Headed in a Bad Direction': Omicron Variant May Bring Second-Largest US Covid Wave," *The Guardian*, July 8, 2022.

9. Kirsty Needham, "Australian PM Says His Government Was Too Optimistic before Omicron Surge." *Reuters*, February 1, 2022, sec. Asia Pacific, https://www.reuters.com/markets/funds/australian-pm-outline-a2-billion-research-boost-2022-01-31/.

10. June-Ho Kim, Julia Ah-Reum An, SeungJu Jackie Oh, Juhwan Oh, and Jong-Koo Lee, "Emerging COVID-19 Success Story: South Korea Learned the Lessons of MERS," Our World in Data, 2021, https://ourworldindata.org/covid-exemplar-south-korea.

11. Emma Willoughby, "An Ideal Public Health Model? Vietnam's State-Led, Preventative, Low-Cost Response to COVID-19," *Brookings* (blog), June 29, 2021, https://www.brookings.edu/blog/order-from-chaos/2021/06/29/an-ideal-public-health-model-vietnams-state-led-preventative-low-cost-response-to-covid-19/.

12. Blake Hereth, Paul Tubig, Ashton Sorrels, Anna Muldoon, Kelly Hills, and Nicholas G. Evans, "Long Covid and Disability: A Brave New World," *BMJ* (in press).

13. George J. Annas, "Bioterrorism and Public Health Law," *JAMA* 288, no. 21 (December 4, 2002): 2685–2685, https://doi.org/10.1001/jama.288.21.2685-JLT1204

-2-1; George J. Annas, "Bioterrorism, Public Health, and Civil Liberties," *New England Journal of Medicine* 346, no. 17 (April 25, 2002): 1337–1342, https://doi.org/10.1056 /NEJM200204253461722; George J. Annas, "Bioterrorism, Public Health, and Human Rights," *Health Affairs* 21, no. 6 (November 1, 2002): 94–97, https://doi.org/10.1377 /hlthaff.21.6.94; Lawrence O. Gostin, "Public Health Law in an Age of Terrorism: Rethinking Individual Rights and Common Goods," *Health Affairs* 21, no. 6 (November 2002): 79–93, https://doi.org/10.1377/hlthaff.21.6.79; Lawrence O. Gostin et al., "The Model State Emergency Health Powers Act: Planning for and Response to Bioterrorism and Naturally Occurring Infectious Diseases," *JAMA* 288, no. 5 (August 7, 2002): 622–628, https://doi.org/10.1001/jama.288.5.622; James G. Hodge, "Bioterrorism Law and Policy: Critical Choices in Public Health," *Journal of Law, Medicine & Ethics* 30, no. 2 (2002): 254–261, https://doi.org/10.1111/j.1748-720X.2002.tb00391.x; G. J. Annas, "Blinded by Bioterrorism: Public Health and Liberty in the 21st Century," *Health Matrix*, 2003, http://heinonline.org/hol-cgi-bin/get_pdf.cgi?handle=hein.journals /hmax13&section=8; George J. Annas, "Puppy Love: Bioterrorism, Civil Rights, and Public Health Dunwody Commentary," *Florida Law Review* 55, no. 5 (2003): 1171–1190; Lawrence O. Gostin, "When Terrorism Threatens Health: How Far Are Limitations on Personal and Economic Liberties Justified," *Florida Law Review*, 2003, http://heinonline .org/hol-cgi-bin/get_pdf.cgi?handle=hein.journals/uflr55&section=59; Lawrence O. Gostin, "The Model State Emergency Health Powers Act: Public Health and Civil Liberties in a Time of Terrorism," *Health Matrix: Journal of Law-Medicine* 13, no. 1 (Winter 2003): 3; Lawrence O. Gostin, "When Terrorism Threatens Health: How Far Are Limitations on Human Rights Justified," *Journal of Law, Medicine & Ethics* 31, no. 4 (December 1, 2003): 524–528, https://doi.org/10.1111/j.1748-720X.2003.tb00120.x; Lawrence O. Gostin, "When Terrorism Threatens Health: How Far Are Limitations on Personal and Economic Liberties Justified Dunwody Distinguished Lecture in Law," *Florida Law Review* 55, no. 5 (2003): 1105–1170; J. M. Haas, "Addressing Bioterrorism. What Ethical Issues and Questions Surround Potential Responses to Bioterrorist Attacks?," *Healthcare Executive* 18, no. 3 (2003): 76–79; W. E. Parmet, "Quarantine Redux: Bioterrorism, AIDS and the Curtailment of Individual Liberty in the Name of Public Health," *Health Matrix*, 2003, http://heinonline.org/hol-cgi-bin/get_pdf.cgi?handle=hein.journals/hmax13 &section=10; Victoria Sutton, "A Multidisciplinary Approach to an Ethic of Biodefense and Bioterrorism," *Journal of Law, Medicine & Ethics* 33, no. 2 (June 2005): 310–322, https://doi.org/10.1111/j.1748-720X.2005.tb00496.x; Michael Gross, *Bioethics and Armed Conflict: Moral Dilemmas of Medicine and War* (Cambridge, MA: MIT Press, 2006), http://books.google.com/books?id=7ik3AgAAQBAJ&printsec=frontcover&dq=michael +gross+modern+military+bioethics&hl=&cd=3&source=gbs_api; J. Watkins, "Bioterrorism: Cases When Public Health Agencies Should Have Sweeping Powers," *Internet Journal of Allied Health Sciences and Practice*, 2006, http://nsuworks.nova.edu/ijahsp/vol4 /iss2/8/; George J. Annas, "Bioterrorism, Public Health, and Civil Liberties," *Dx.Doi. Org.Libproxy.Uml.Edu* 346, no. 17 (October 2009): 1337–1342, https://doi.org/10.1056 /NEJM200204253461722; Christian Enemark, *Biosecurity Dilemmas: Dreaded Diseases,*

Ethical Responses, and the Health of Nations (Washington, DC: Georgetown University Press, 2017).

14. Enemark, *Biosecurity Dilemmas*; Nicholas Greig Evans and Michael J. Selgelid, "Biosecurity and Open-Source Biology: The Promise and Peril of Distributed Synthetic Biological Technologies," *Science and Engineering Ethics* 21, no. 4 (September 2014): 1065–1083, https://doi.org/10.1007/s11948-014-9591-3; Nicholas Greig Evans, Marc Lipsitch, and Meira Levinson, "The Ethics of Biosafety Considerations in Gain-of-Function Research Resulting in the Creation of Potential Pandemic Pathogens," *Journal of Medical Ethics* 41, no. 11 (November 2015): 901–908, https://doi.org/10.1136/medethics-2014-102619; Nicholas Greig Evans, "Ebola: From Public Health Crisis to National Security Threat," in *Biological Threats in the 21st Century*, ed. Filippa Lentzos (London: Imperial College Press, 2016), 277–292, https://doi.org/10.1142/9781783269488_0017; Nicholas Greig Evans, "Ethical and Philosophical Considerations for Gain-of-Function Policy: The Importance of Alternate Experiments," *Frontiers in Bioengineering and Biotechnology* 6 (February 2018): e1875, https://doi.org/10.3389/fbioe.2018.00011; Nicholas Greig Evans and Thomas Inglesby, "Biosecurity and Public Health Ethics Issues Raised by Biological Threats," in *The Oxford Handbook of Public Health Ethics*, ed. Anna C. Mastroianni, Jeffrey P. Kahn, and Nancy E. Kass (Oxford: Oxford University Press, 2019), 773–785, https://doi.org/10.1093/oxfordhb/9780190245191.013.67.

15. Evans and Inglesby, "Biosecurity and Public Health Ethics Issues," https://doi.org/10.1093/oxfordhb/9780190245191.013.67.

16. In addition to being the received view of public health ethics for many, this is also a nod to the debate between the "orthodox" and "revisionists" in the ethics of armed conflict.

17. James F. Childress et al., "Public Health Ethics: Mapping the Terrain," *Journal of Law, Medicine & Ethics* 30, no. 2 (June 2002): 170–178, https://doi.org/10.1111/j.1748-720X.2002.tb00384.x.

18. See, e.g., A. M. Viens, Cécile M. Bensimon, and Ross E. G. Upshur, "Your Liberty or Your Life: Reciprocity in the Use of Restrictive Measures in Contexts of Contagion," *Journal of Bioethical Inquiry* 6, no. 2 (June 2009): 207–217, https://doi.org/10.1007/s11673-009-9149-2; Michael J. Selgelid, "A Moderate Pluralist Approach to Public Health Policy and Ethics," *Public Health Ethics* 2, no. 2 (August 2009): 195–205, https://doi.org/10.1093/phe/php018; Timothy Allen and Michael J. Selgelid, "Necessity and Least Infringement Conditions in Public Health Ethics," *Medicine, Health Care and Philosophy* 51 (April 2017): 525–535, https://doi.org/10.1007/s11019-017-9775-0.

19. Childress et al., "Mapping the Terrain," 170–171.

20. Childress et al., "Mapping the Terrain," 172.

21. "The Model State Emergency Health Powers Act," 6:n9.

22. World Health Organization, "International Health Regulations–3rd Ed." (Geneva, Switzerland: WHO, 2005), 20. Emphasis added.

23. WHO, "International Health Regulations," 29. Emphasis added.

24. World Health Organization, "Global Health Ethics: Key Issues" (Geneva, Switzerland: World Health Organization, 2015), https://apps.who.int/iris/bitstream/handle/10665/164576/9789240694033_eng.pdf?sequence=1.

25. International Commission of Jurists, "Siracusa Principles on the Limitation and Derogation Provisions in the International Covenant on Civil and Political Rights," 1985, §10–11. See Allen and Selgelid, "Necessity and Least Infringement Conditions," 528.

26. Alan O. Sykes, "The Least Restrictive Means," *University of Chicago Law Review* 70, no. 1 (2003): 403.

27. Jonathan D. Moreno, *In the Wake of Terror: Medicine and Morality in a Time of Crisis* (Cambridge, MA: MIT Press, 2003), 19.

28. See John Tobin, "The Right to Health and Health Related Human Rights," in *Foundations of Global Health and Human Rights*, ed. Lawrence O. Gostin and Benjamin Mason Meier (Oxford: Oxford University Press, 2020), 73; Flavia Bustreo and Curtis F. J. Doebbler, "The Rights Based Approach to Health," in *Foundations of Global Health and Human Rights*, ed. Lawrence O. Gostin and Benjamin Mason Meier (Oxford: Oxford University Press, 2020), 90–92; George J. Annas, *Worst Case Bioethics: Death, Disaster, and Public Health* (New York: Oxford University Press, 2010), 187.

29. R. Bayer, C. Levine, and S. M. Wolf, "HIV Antibody Screening. An Ethical Framework for Evaluating Proposed Programs," *JAMA* 256, no. 13 (October 3, 1986): 1768–1774, https://doi.org/10.1001/jama.256.13.1768.

30. Stefan Elbe, "Should HIV/AIDS Be Securitized? The Ethical Dilemmas of Linking HIV/AIDS and Security," *International Studies Quarterly* 50, no. 1 (March 1, 2006): 119–144, https://doi.org/10.1111/j.1468-2478.2006.00395.x; Dan W. Brock and Daniel Wikler, "Ethical Challenges In Long-Term Funding For HIV/AIDS," *Health Affairs* 28, no. 6 (November 1, 2009): 1666–1676, https://doi.org/10.1377/hlthaff.28.6.1666; Lauren M. Broyles, Alison M. Colbert, and Judith A. Erlen, "Medication Practice and Feminist Thought: A Theoretical and Ethical Response to Adherence in Hiv/Aids," *Bioethics* 19, no. 4 (2005): 362–378, https://doi.org/10.1111/j.1467-8519.2005.00449.x.

31. Hodge and Gostin in Moreno, 19.

32. For those commentaries see Lawrence O. Gostin, "Public Health, Ethics, and Human Rights: A Tribute to the Late Jonathan Mann," *Journal of Law, Medicine & Ethics: A Journal of the American Society of Law, Medicine & Ethics* 29, no. 2 (2001):

121–130, https://doi.org/10.1111/j.1748-720x.2001.tb00330.x; J. M. Mann, "Medicine and Public Health, Ethics and Human Rights." *The Hastings Center Report* 27, no. 3 (June 1997): 6–13.

For a philosophical grounding of human rights, see John Kleinig and Nicholas Greig Evans. "Human Flourishing, Human Dignity, and Human Rights." *Law and Philosophy* 32, no. 5 (September 2013): 539–564.

33. Steven H. Miles, "Abu Ghraib: Its Legacy for Military Medicine," *The Lancet* 364, no. 9435 (August 2004): 725–729, https://doi.org/10.1016/S0140-6736(04)16902-X; *Oath Betrayed: America's Torture Doctors* (Berkeley: University of California Press, 2009); Nicholas Greig Evans, D. A. Sisti, and Jonathan D. Moreno, "Ethical Considerations on the Complicity of Psychologists and Scientists in Torture," *Journal of the Royal Army Medical Corps* 165, no. 4 (February 2019): 248–255, https://doi.org/10.1136/jramc-2018-001008.

34. Annas, "Puppy Love."

35. Annas, "Puppy Love."

36. Jens David Ohlin, and Larry May, *Necessity in International Law* (New York: Oxford University Press, 2016).

37. Rebecca Haffajee, Wendy E. Parmet, and Michelle M. Mello, "What Is a Public Health 'Emergency'?," *New England Journal of Medicine* 371, no. 11 (September 11, 2014): 988, https://doi.org/10.1056/NEJMp1406167.

38. Annas, *Worst Case Bioethics*.

39. George J. Annas, "Bioterrorism, Public Health, And Human Rights," *Health Affairs* 21, no. 6 (November 1, 2002): 96.

40. George J. Annas, "Bioterrorism, Public Health, and Civil Liberties," *New England Journal of Medicine* 346, no. 17 (April 25, 2002): 1339.

41. Annas, "Bioterrorism, Public Health, and Civil Liberties," 1340.

42. Gostin, "When Terrorism Threatens Health: How Far Are Limitations on Personal and Economic Liberties Justified," 1108.

43. Gostin, "Public Health Law in An Age of Terrorism," 88.

44. James F. Childress and Ruth Gaare Bernheim, "Beyond the Liberal and Communitarian Impasse: A Framework and Vision for Public Health," *Florida Law Review* 55, no. 5 (2003): 1191–1291.

45. Gostin, "When Terrorism Threatens Health: How Far Are Limitations on Human Rights Justified," 525.

46. Gostin, "When Terrorism Threatens Health: How Far Are Limitations on Human Rights Justified," 524. Annas locates the change for Gostin in his work with the US

CDC beginning in 2001 after the anthrax attacks. See Annas, "Puppy Love." But whatever the reason, it is clear that Gostin retains some of his views on rights, albeit in a restrictive form.

47. Hodge Jr. and Gostin, "Protecting the Public's Health in an Era of Bioterrorism," 19.

48. Hodge Jr. and Gostin, "Protecting the Public's Health in an Era of Bioterrorism," 24.

49. Allen and Selgelid, "Necessity and Least Infringement Conditions," 532.

50. UN Universal Declaration of Human Rights, art. 29(2). Benjamin Mason Meier, Thérèse Murphy, and Lawrence O. Gostin, "The Birth and Development of Human Rights for Health," in *Foundations of Global Health and Human Rights*, ed. Benjamin Mason Meier and Lawrence O. Gostin (New York: Oxford University Press), 35.

51. See, e.g., Childress and Bernheim, "Beyond the Liberal and Communitarian Impasse"; Wendy E. Parmet, "Liberalism, Communitarianism, and Public Health: Comments on Lawrence O. Gostin's Lecture Dunwody Commentary," *Florida Law Review* 55, no. 5 (2003): 1221–1240.

52. Philip Pettit provides a consequentialist account of rights that acknowledges that we may think about the costs of respecting rights, but only in a restrictive view wherein we must think not only about the trade-off between rights and utility but include the trade-off wherein we live with the knowledge that our rights are vulnerable to this kind of calculation. See Philip Pettit, "The Consequentialist Can Recognise Rights," *Philosophical Quarterly* 38, no. 150 (January 1988): 42–55, https://doi.org/10.2307/2220266.

53. An example of a framework that achieves something similar can be found in R. E. G. Upshur, "Principles for the Justification of Public Health Intervention," *Canadian Journal of Public Health—Revue Canadienne de Santé Publique* 93, no. 2 (March 2002): 101–103, https://doi.org/10.1007/BF03404547

54. Bustreo and Doebbler, "The Rights Based Approach to Health," 73.

55. Jim Childress, in more recent work, has categorized his view as broadly "presumptivist." See James F. Childress, *Public Bioethics: Principles and Problems* (Oxford: Oxford University Press, 2020), 252–272. This view is broadly supported by a variety of scholars; e.g., James Griffin, *On Human Rights* (Oxford: Oxford University Press, 2009); Kleinig and Evans, "Human Flourishing."

56. Childress et. al, "Mapping the Terrain," 172–174.

57. Amy L. Fairchild and Ronald Bayer, "Ethics and the Conduct of Public Health Surveillance," *Science* 303, no. 5658 (January 2004): 631–632, https://doi.org/10.1126/science.1094038.

58. George J. Annas, "Control of Tuberculosis—The Law and the Public's Health," *New England Journal of Medicine* 328, no. 8 (February 25, 1993): 586; Mark McClellan et al., "A National COVID-19 Surveillance System: Achieving Containment" (Duke

Margolis Center for Health Policy, April 7, 2020), 9; Upshur, "Principles for the Justification of Public Health Intervention," 102; Lawrence O. Gostin and Madison Powers, "What Does Social Justice Require for The Public's Health? Public Health Ethics and Policy Imperatives," *Health Affairs* 25, no. 4 (July 1, 2006): 1059.

59. Childress et al., "Mapping the Terrain."

60. Nancy E. Kass, "An Ethics Framework for Public Health," *American Journal of Public Health* 91, no. 11 (November 2001): 1776–1782.

61. Nancy E. Kass and Andrea Carlson Gielen, "The Ethics of Contact Tracing Programs and Their Implications for Women," *Duke Journal of Gender Law & Policy* 5, no. 1 (1998): 89–102.

62. The National Commission for the Protection of Human Subjects of Biomedical and Behavioral Research, "Ethical Principles and Guidelines for the Protection of Human Subjects of Research" (Washington, DC: Department of Health, Education, and Welfare, April 1979), https://www.hhs.gov/ohrp/sites/default/files/the-belmont -report-508c_FINAL.pdf.

63. Gostin, "When Terrorism Threatens Health: How Far Are Limitations on Personal and Economic Liberties Justified," 1107. Note that there is a paper of the same name produced in the *Journal of Law Medicine and Ethics*; this as I understand it is a précis of the *Florida Law Review* article.

64. Gostin, "When Terrorism Threatens Health: How Far Are Limitations on Personal and Economic Liberties Justified," n.195, 1141–1145.

65. Gostin, "When Terrorism Threatens Health: How Far Are Limitations on Personal and Economic Liberties Justified," 1146.

66. Robert Nozick, *Anarchy, State, and Utopia* (New York: Basic Books, 1974), ch. 1.

67. Nozick, *Anarchy, State, and Utopia*, 110n.

68. Michael Davis has an excellent essay on why Nozick *should* be committed to the welfare state; but he acknowledges that Nozick himself and most libertarians would reject that position even at the risk of incoherence. See Michael Davis, "Nozick's Argument for the Legitimacy of the Welfare State." *Ethics* 97, no. 3 (April 1987): 576–594, https://doi.org/10.2307/2381180?ref=search-gateway:1ca25a54392455b1e7b50f57d8b 21e77.

69. Gostin, "When Terrorism Threatens Health: How Far Are Limitations on Personal and Economic Liberties Justified," 1148.

70. Gostin, "When Terrorism Threatens Health: How Far Are Limitations on Personal and Economic Liberties Justified," 1148.

71. Norman Daniels, *Just Health: Meeting Health Needs Fairly* (Cambridge: Cambridge University Press, 2007).

72. Griffin Trotter, *The Ethics of Coercion in Mass Casualty Medicine* (Baltimore, MD: Johns Hopkins University Press, 2007). Trotter, in conversation at the American Society for Bioethics and Humanities 2014 Annual Conference in San Diego, informed me that he was certainly not Nozickian in a strict sense, but rather more sympathetic to the work of Tristram Englehardt Jr. who, however, is a libertarian about rights in much the same way as Nozick. While Englehardt's libertarianism is often seen as repugnant even by other libertarians in bioethics, this is typically in terms of his treatment of vulnerable groups such as the disabled as nonpersons rather than for public health reasons I discuss here. See, e.g., Sigrid Fry-Revere, "A Libertarian Critique of H. Tristram Engelhardt, Jr.'s 'The Foundations of Bioethics,'" *Journal of Clinical Ethics* 3, no. 1 (1992): 46–52.

73. Herington, Dawson, and Draper, "Obesity."

74. Lawrence O. Gostin, "Another Voice: Public Health Emergencies: What Counts?," *The Hastings Center Report* 44, no. 6 (2014): 36.

75. Nick Bostrom, *Superintelligence: Paths, Dangers, Strategies* (Oxford: Oxford University Press, 2014).

76. Michael J. Selgelid, "A Moderate Pluralist Approach to Public Health Policy and Ethics," *Public Health Ethics* 2, no. 2 (August 2009): 195–205, https://doi.org/10.1093/phe/php018.

77. Marc Lipsitch, Nicholas Greig Evans, and Owen Cotton Barratt, "Underprotection of Unpredictable Statistical Lives Compared to Predictable Ones," *Risk Analysis*, July 2016, https://doi.org/10.1111/risa.12658.

78. This is not to say that mistakenly being one death shy of the "limit" for violating rights would be the same as being 1,000 deaths shy. Rather, the serious wrong a rights infringement represents here is such that we need to be particularly confident in the consequences before we act. Here, I'm separating out the criterion for ranking states of affairs from the cognitive process by which we judge which states of affairs to pursue. See, e.g., Pettit, "Consequentialist."

79. Frederick Schauer, "Slippery Slopes," *Harvard Law Review* 99, no. 2 (1985): 366–367.

80. Fritz Allhoff, Nicholas Greig Evans, and Adam Henschke, "Not Just Wars: Expansions and Alternatives to the Just War Tradition," in *Children of Capital: Eugenics in the World of Private Biotechnology*, ed. Fritz Allhoff and Adam Henschke (New York: Routledge, 2013), 1–8.

81. P. Foot, "The Problem of Abortion and the Doctrine of the Double Effect," in *Virtues and Vices and Other Essays in Moral Philosophy* (New York: Oxford University Press, 1993), 19–32.

82. Daniel P. Sulmasy and Edmund D. Pellegrino, "The Rule of Double Effect: Clearing Up the Double Talk," *Archives of Internal Medicine* 159, no. 6 (March 22, 1999): 545–550, https://doi.org/10.1001/archinte.159.6.545.

83. Both Walzer and May have excellent prehistories of just war theory. See Michael Walzer, *Just and Unjust Wars: A Moral Argument with Historical Illustrations* (New York: Basic Books, 2015); Larry May, *Contingent Pacifism: Revisiting Just War Theory* (Cambridge: Cambridge University Press, 2015), ch. 1–2.

84. Centers for Disease Control and Prevention, "SARS, CDC Guidance Supplement D: Community Containment Measures, Including Non-Hospital Isolation and Quarantine," February 8, 2019, https://www.cdc.gov/sars/guidance/d-quarantine/community .html.

85. CDC, "SARS, CDC Guidance Supplement D."

86. Gerhard Øverland, "High-Fliers: Who Should Bear the Risk of Humanitarian Intervention?," in *New Wars and New Soldiers*, ed. Paolo Tripodi and Jessica Wolfendale (Surrey, UK: Ashgate Publishing, 2011), 69–86.

87. I appreciate the feedback of one of the reviewers of an early version of this project for this feedback.

88. See, e.g., L. Alexander, "Deontology at the Threshold," *San Diego Law Review* 37 (2000): 893–912; Samuel Scheffler, *The Rejection of Consequentialism: A Philosophical Investigation of the Considerations Underlying Rival Moral Conceptions* (Oxford: Oxford University Press, 1994); David Ross, *The Right and the Good*, ed. Philip Stratton-Lake, 2nd ed. (Oxford: Clarendon Press, 2003).

89. Walzer, "Just and Unjust Wars," 254–256.

90. Though cf. David Rodin, *War and Self-Defense* (Oxford: Clarendon Press, 2005); Helen Frowe, *Defensive Killing* (Oxford: Oxford University Press, 2014).

91. Larry May, "Human Rights, Proportionality, and the Lives of Soldiers," in *The Ethics of War*, ed. Saba Bazargan and Samuel C. Rickless (Oxford: Oxford University Press, 2017), 57.

92. James F. Childress, "Just-War Theories: The Bases, Interrelations, Priorities, and Functions of Their Criteria," *Theological Studies* 39, no. 3 (1978): 427–445, https:// doi.org/10.1177/004056397803900302.

93. National Academies of Sciences, Medicine, and Engineering, *Exploring Opportunities in Correctional Health, Law, and Law Enforcement, Integrating Responses at the Intersection of Opioid Use Disorder and Infectious Disease Epidemics: Proceedings of a Workshop* (Washington, DC: National Academies Press, 2018), 104–105.

94. "Just-War Theories," 431–432.

95. See, e.g., Griffin, "On Human Rights," ch. 1.

96. May, "Contingent Pacifism," ch. 3.

Chapter 4

1. *New York Times*, https://www.nytimes.com/2020/10/02/us/politics/trump-covid .html.

2. Pien Huang, "Trump's Missed Opportunities to Personally Stop the Spread of the Coronavirus," NPR.org, October 6, 2020, https://www.npr.org/sections/latest-updates -trump-covid-19-results/2020/10/06/920846471/trumps-missed-opportunities-to-stop -the-spread-of-coronavirus.

3. Dena Grayson, MD, PhD, "‼Even If You Believe the WH's Latest Version of the Timeline, Trump Still *knowingly* Exposed Hundreds of People to the Deadly #coronavirus on Thursday. THAT IS A CRIME. Trump Should Be Charged with Reckless Endangerment, a #felony. #GOPSuperSpreaders #TrumpVirus #TrumpCovid," Tweet, *@DrDenaGrayson* (blog), October 3, 2020, https://twitter.com/DrDenaGrayson /status/1312456861669421057.

4. Anne Margaret Daniel, "It Is a Felony Crime to Expose Others to Communicable Disease in Minnesota: Https://T.Co/BfzweEZndO It Ranges from Misdemeanor to Felony in Ohio: Https://T.Co/SpoVZl5PEF @GovTimWalz and @GovMikeDeWine You Have Grounds for Legal Action. Trump Knew He Had Covid, and Came to You," *Twitter* (blog), October 3, 2020, https://twitter.com/venetianblonde/status /1312432194862944257.

5. John Cusack, "Call on Him to Resign If You Hold Public Office." @brianjtrautman: Absolutely Criminal. Not a Political Matter. It's a Matter of Law and Accountability. Total Insanity. In a Democracy, Trump Would Be Charged with a Violent Felony. #TrumpCovid: Https://T.Co/FS7a56Kog1 Tweet, *@johncusack* (blog), October 3, 2020, https://twitter.com/johncusack/status/1312503640968421377.

6. Barbara Goldberg, "As People Use COVID-19 as Weapon, U.S. States Mull Criminal Crackdowns," *Reuters*, May 14, 2020, https://www.reuters.com/article/us-health -coronavirus-usa-weaponization-idUSKBN22Q1PK.

7. M. Bloom, "How Terrorist Groups Will Try to Capitalize on the Coronavirus Crisis: Just Security," https://www.justsecurity.org/69508/how-terrorist-groups-will -try-to-capitalize-on-the-coronavirus-crisis/. Published April 3, 2020. Accessed October 27, 2020.

8. Paul LeBlanc, "People Intentionally Spreading Coronavirus Could Be Charged with Terrorism, DOJ Says," CNN, accessed December 27, 2020, https://www.cnn .com/2020/03/25/politics/coronavirus-terrorism-justice-department/index.html.

9. US Centers for Disease Control and Prevention, "HIV and STD Criminalization Laws | Law | Policy and Law | HIV/AIDS | CDC," December 21, 2020, https://www.cdc .gov/hiv/policies/law/states/exposure.html.

10. Laura Flanders, "If the President Had HIV He Could Be in Prison," Common Dreams, accessed December 27, 2020, https://www.commondreams.org/views/2020 /10/07/if-president-had-hiv-he-could-be-prison.

11. For a partial rejection of these views, see, e.g., May, *Contingent Pacifism: Revisiting Just War Theory* (Cambridge: Cambridge University Press, 2015).

12. I've already covered much of this in previous chapters, but a partial list of these criticisms includes Kendall Hoyt, *Long Shot: Vaccines for National Defense* (Cambridge, MA: Harvard University Press, 2012), 142–160; Victoria Sutton, "Biodefense: Who's in Charge?," *Health Matrix: Journal of Law-Medicine* 13, no. 1 (Winter 2003): 117; Christian Enemark, "United States Biodefense, International Law, and the Problem of Intent," *Politics and the Life Sciences* 24, no. 1 & 2 (2005): 32–42, https://doi.org/10 .2990/1471-5457(2005)24[32:usbila]2.0.co;2; Enemark, *Biosecurity Dilemmas*, 139–156; Stefan Elbe, *Pandemics, Pills, and Politics: Governing Global Health Security* (Baltimore, MD: Johns Hopkins University Press, 2018); Anne Roemer-Mahler and Stefan Elbe, "The Race for Ebola Drugs: Pharmaceuticals, Security and Global Health Governance," *Third World Quarterly* 37, no. 3 (March 3, 2016): 487–506, https://doi.org/10.1080 /01436597.2015.1111136; Frank Smith and Frank L. Smith III, *American Biodefense: How Dangerous Ideas about Biological Weapons Shape National Security* (Ithaca, NY: Cornell University Press, 2014).

13. Cf. Enemark, *Biosecurity Dilemmas*; Herrington, "The Concept of Security"; Selgelid and Enemark, "Infectious Diseases, Security, and Ethics."

14. Weir, "Inventing Global Health Security, 1994–2005."

15. David Fidler, "Microbialpolitik: Infectious Diseases and International Relations," *American University International Law Review* 14 (January 1, 1998): 1–53.

16. Margaret P. Battin, Leslie P. Francis, Jay A. Jacobson, and Charles B. Smith, *The Patient as Victim and Vector: Ethics and Infectious Disease* (Oxford: Oxford University Press, 2008).

17. See, e.g., Herington, "The Concept of Security."

18. https://www.unaids.org/en/resources/fact-sheet.

19. World Health Organization (WHO), Global Status Report on Road Safety 2018, December 2018, accessed October 28, 2020, https://www.who.int/violence_injury _prevention/road_safety_status/2018/en/.

20. W. S. Hotchkiss, "The American Medical Association and the War on AIDS," *Public Health Reports* 103, no. 3 (1988): 282–288.

21. Many thanks to Lance Wahlert for pointing this out to me in conversation.

22. See, e.g., Debbie Nathan and Michael Snedeker, *Satan's Silence: Ritual Abuse and The Making of a Modern American Witch Hunt* (New York: Basic Books, 1995). For

those interested in a reliable and free history, drawn in part from Nathan and Sne-deker's book, see, e.g., Robert Evans, "Part One: The Satanic Panic: America's First QAnon," Behind the Bastards, accessed December 27, 2020, https://www.iheart.com /podcast/105-behind-the-bastards-29236323/episode/part-one-the-satanic-panic -americas-73004015/.

23. Anders Wimo et al., "The Worldwide Costs of Dementia 2015 and Comparisons with 2010," *Alzheimer's & Dementia* 13, no. 1 (January 1, 2017): 1–7, https://doi.org/10 .1016/j.jalz.2016.07.150.

24. Michael Moehler, "In Defense of a Democratic Productivist Welfare State," *European Journal of Philosophy* 25, no. 2 (June 2017): 416–439, https://doi.org/10.1111 /ejop.12157.

25. G. Dennis Shanks,and John F. Brundage, "Pathogenic Responses among Young Adults during the 1918 Influenza Pandemic," *Emerging Infectious Diseases* 18 (2012): 201–207, https://doi:10.3201/eid1802.102042.

26. Akilah Johnson and Nina Martin, "How COVID-19 Hollowed Out a Generation of Young Black Men" *ProPublica*, December 22, 2020, accessed June 8, 2022, https:// www.propublica.org/article/how-covid-19-hollowed-out-a-generation-of-young -black-men.

27. *Jacobson v. Massachusetts*, 197 U.S. 11 (1904), periodical, https://www.loc.gov /item/usrep197011/.

28. Gerhard Øverland, Gerhard. "Conditional Threats." *Journal of Moral Philosophy* 7, no. 3 (2010): 334–345, https://doi.org/10.1163/174552410X511400.

29. Walzer, *Just and Unjust Wars*, 30–33.

30. See, e.g., Seth Lazar, "War's End and the Structure of Just War Theory" in *The Ethics of War*, ed. Saba Bazargan-Forward and Samuel C. Rickless (New York: Oxford University Press, 2017).

31. Judith Jarvis Thomson, "Self-Defense," *Philosophy & Public Affairs* 20 (1991): 283–310, 287; Jeff McMahan, "Innocence, Self-Defense and Killing in War." *Journal of Political Philosophy* 2, no. 3 (1994): 193–221, https://doi.org/10.1111/j.1467-9760.1994 .tb00021.x.

32. Paul B. Larsen, "Asteroid Legal Regime: Time for a Change," *Journal of Space Law* 39, no. 2 (2013): 275–326.

33. Youde also uses this term, albeit in a slightly different sense. See his *Global Health Governance*, 139–145.

34. Nicholas Greig Evans, "Ebola: From Public Health Crisis to National Security Threat."

35. The other significant work here is Selgelid's "Ethics and Infectious Disease."

36. Battin et al., 90.

37. Battin et al., 90.

38. Battin et al., 107.

39. If this sounds overly paranoid, I invite you to ask an epidemiologist what they think about raw sprouts, or oysters. It may be paranoid, but less uncommon than you might think.

40. Battin et al., ch. 1.

41. Battin et al., 158–159.

42. Battin et al., 322.

43. Jeff McMahan, "Who Is Morally Liable to Be Killed in War," *Analysis* 71, no. 3 (July 1, 2011): 544–559; Jeff McMahan, *The Ethics of Killing: Problems at the Margins of Life* (New York: Oxford University Press, 2002).

44. McMahan, "Innocence, Self-Defense and Killing in War," 388.

45. McMahan, "Innocence, Self-Defense and Killing in War," 388.

46. This is a core component to Helen Frowe's revision to the tradition. See Helen Frowe, *Defensive Killing* (Oxford: Oxford University Press, 2014).

47. Philip Pettit, "The Consequentialist Can Recognise Rights," *Philosophical Quarterly* 38, no. 150 (January 1988): 42–55, https://doi.org/10.2307/2220266; Philip Pettit, "Consequentialism and Respect for Persons," *Ethics* 100, no. 1 (October 1989): 116–126, https://doi.org/10.2307/2381149?ref=search-gateway:f6dfa0368177ed4f28 320943db714f48; Philip Pettit, *Republicanism: A Theory of Freedom and Government* (Oxford: Oxford University Press, 1997), https://www.oxfordscholarship.com/view /10.1093/0198296428.001.0001/acprof-9780198296423.

48. For more on proportionate means, see, e.g., Helen Frowe, *Defensive Killing* (Oxford: Oxford University Press, 2014).

49. Most theories, I suspect, agree with this. In consequentialist theories this is simply the inverse of Singer's famous argument about failing to benefit someone when I could do so easily. Peter Singer, "Famine, Affluence, and Morality," *Philosophy & Public Affairs* 1, no. 3 (1972): 229–243.

For deontologists, this is captured by Lazar's work in which he described how imposing additional risk of harm can fail by more grievously undervaluing his standing and interests, and more seriously undermining his security by exposing a disposition to harm him across all counterfactual scenarios in which the probability of killing an innocent person is that high or less. Seth Lazar, "Risky Killing," *Journal of Moral Philosophy* (February 2017): 1–26, https://doi.org/10.1163/17455243-46810076.

50. David Rodin, *War and Self-Defense* (Oxford: Clarendon Press, 2005).

51. Michael G. Rossmann and Venigalla B. Rao, "Viruses: Sophisticated Biological Machines," *Advances in Experimental Medicine and Biology* 726 (2012): 1–3, https://doi .org/10.1007/978-1-4614-0980-9_1.

52. May, "Contingent Pacifism."

53. Saba Bazargan-Forward, "Varieties of Contingent Pacifism in War," SSRN Scholarly Paper (Rochester, NY: Social Science Research Network, 2012), https://papers .ssrn.com/abstract=2914686.

54. May, "Contingent Pacifism."

55. Crystal Franco et al., "The National Disaster Medical System: Past, Present, and Suggestions for the Future," *Biosecurity and Bioterrorism: Biodefense Strategy, Practice, and Science* 5, no. 4 (December 1, 2007): 319–326.

56. Donald A. Henderson et al., "A Plague on Your City: Observations from TOPOFF," *Clinical Infectious Diseases* 32, no. 3 (February 1, 2001): 436–445, https://doi.org/10 .1086/318513.

57. See, e.g., the recommendations in Tara O'Toole, Mair Michael, and Thomas V. Inglesby, "Shining Light on 'Dark Winter,'" *Clinical Infectious Diseases* 34, no. 7 (April 1, 2002): 972–983, https://doi.org/10.1086/339909.

58. Franco et al., "The National Disaster Medical System."

59. Luciana Borio, "21st Century Pandemic, Prehistoric Clinical Trials," BioCentury, June 26, 2020, https://www.biocentury.com/article/305565/21st-century-pandemic -prehistoric-clinical-trials.

60. Amy Maxmen and Jeff Tollefson, "Two Decades of Pandemic War Games Failed to Account for Donald Trump," *Nature* 584 (2020): 26–29, https://doi:10.1038/d41586 -020-02277-6.

61. Talha Burki, "The Origin of SARS-CoV-2," *The Lancet Infectious Diseases* 20, no. 9 (September 1, 2020): 1018–1019, https://doi.org/10.1016/S1473-3099(20)30641-1.

62. Kurt J. Vandegrift et al., "Ecology of Avian Influenza Viruses in a Changing World," *Annals of the New York Academy of Sciences* 1195 (May 2010): 113–128, https://doi.org /10.1111/j.1749-6632.2010.05451.x.

63. Andrew P. Dobson et al., "Ecology and Economics for Pandemic Prevention," *Science* 369, no. 6502 (July 24, 2020): 379–381, https://doi.org/10.1126/science.abc3189; Jesús Olivero et al., "Recent Loss of Closed Forests Is Associated with Ebola Virus Disease Outbreaks," *Scientific Reports* 7, no. 1 (October 30, 2017): 14291, https://doi.org/10.1038 /s41598-017-14727-9.

64. Sadie J. Ryan et al., "Global Expansion and Redistribution of Aedes-Borne Virus Transmission Risk with Climate Change," *PLOS Neglected Tropical Diseases* 13, no. 3 (March 28, 2019): e0007213, https://doi.org/10.1371/journal.pntd.0007213.

65. Kim Yi Dionne and Laura Seay, "8. American Perceptions of Africa during an Ebola Outbreak," in *Ebola's Message* (PubPub, 2020), https://covid-19.mitpress.mit.edu/pub/ialzqbqw/release/1.

66. Nicholas G. Evans, Tara Smith, and Maimuna S. Majumder, "Ebola's Message: A Multidisciplinary Call to Action," in *Ebola's Message* (PubPub, 2020), https://covid-19.mitpress.mit.edu/pub/mq0e3o9g/release/1; Chernoh Alpha M. Bah, *The Ebola Outbreak in West Africa: Corporate Gangsters, Multinationals, and Rogue Politicians* (Philadelphia, PA: Africanist Press, 2015).

67. Nicholas G. Evans, Kelly Hills, and Adam C. Levine, "How Should the WHO Guide Access and Benefit Sharing during Infectious Disease Outbreaks?," *AMA Journal of Ethics* 22, no. 1 (January 1, 2020): 28–35, https://doi.org/10.1001/amajethics.2020.28.

68. United Nations, "Describing COVID-19 Pandemic as Wake-Up Call, Dress Rehearsal for Future Challenges, Secretary-General Opens Annual General Assembly Debate with Vision for Solidarity | Meetings Coverage and Press Releases," accessed December 27, 2020, https://www.un.org/press/en/2020/ga12268.doc.htm.

69. "That Mitchell and Webb Look," Season 1 Episode 1, https://youtu.be/rWvpvlT9pJU.

70. There is a military ethics analogy here, but for the sake of brevity I won't cash it out. Jonathan Quong, however, has mounted an argument as to why individuals being shot at by a just attacker might be justified in shooting back. I take it that there is a similar argument that even if we are in some way liable to harm against disease, we aren't simply obligated to lie down and accept our fate.

71. Liang Wang et al., "Inference of Person-to-Person Transmission of COVID-19 Reveals Hidden Super-Spreading Events during the Early Outbreak Phase," *Nature Communications* 11, no. 1 (October 6, 2020): 5006, https://doi.org/10.1038/s41467-020-18836-4.

72. Wang et al., "Inference of Person-to-Person Transmission of COVID-19."

73. Michael Worobey et al., "1970s and 'Patient 0' HIV-1 Genomes Illuminate Early HIV/AIDS History in North America," *Nature* 539, no. 7627 (November 3, 2016): 98–101, https://doi.org/10.1038/nature19827.

74. See Lazar, *Sparing Civilians*, ch. 4.

75. Farah and Farah, "Sick Days in America," 2020, https://farahandfarah.com/studies/sick-days-in-america/.

76. J. Michael McGinnis and William H. Foege, "Actual Causes of Death in the United States," *JAMA* 270, no. 18 (November 10, 1993): 2207–2212, https://doi.org/10.1001/jama.1993.03510180077038.

77. M. G. Marmot et al., "Employment Grade and Coronary Heart Disease in British Civil Servants," *Journal of Epidemiology and Community Health* 32, no. 4 (December 1978): 244–249.

78. Anne Barnhill and Tyler Doggett, "Food Ethics I: Food Production and Food Justice, *Philosophy Compass* 13, no. 3 (March 2018): e12479. See also Lawrence O. Gostin, "Another Voice: Public Health Emergencies: What Counts?" *The Hastings Center Report* 44 (2014): 36.

79. See Danielle M. Wenner, "Nondomination and the Limits of Relational Autonomy," *IJFAB: International Journal of Feminist Approaches to Bioethics 13 (*2020): 28–48.

80. See David Rodin, "The Lesser Evil Obligation," in *The Ethics of War*, ed. Saba Bazargan and Samuel C. Rickless (Oxford University Press, 2017), 28–45.

Chapter 5

1. Or at least, wars that are not civil wars—though even then, civil wars are often fought against the state.

2. Seth Lazar, "War's Endings and the Structure of Just War Theory," in *The Ethics of War*, ed. Saba Bazargan and Samuel C. Rickless (Oxford University Press, 2017), 227–242.

3. James G. Hodge Jr. and Lawrence O. Gostin, "Protecting the Public's Health in an Era of Bioterrorism: The Model State Emergency Health Powers Act," in *In the Wake of Terror: Medicine and Morality in a Time of Crisis*, ed. Jonathan D. Moreno (Cambridge, MA: MIT Press, 2003), 19.

4. Allyn L. Taylor, Roojin Habibi, Gian Luca Burci, Stephanie Dagron, Mark Eccleston-Turner, Lawrence O. Gostin, Benjamin Mason Meier, et al., "Solidarity in the Wake of COVID-19: Reimagining the International Health Regulations," *The Lancet* 396, no. 10244 (July 2020): 82–83, https://doi.org/10.1016/S0140-6736(20)31417-3; Roojin Habibi, Gian Luca Burci, Thana C. de Campos, Danwood Chirwa, Margherita Cinà, Stéphanie Dagron, Mark Eccleston-Turner, et al., "Do Not Violate the International Health Regulations during the COVID-19 Outbreak," *The Lancet* 395, no. 10225 (February 2020): 664–666, https://doi.org/10.1016/S0140-6736(20)30373-1; Jeremy R. Youde, *Global Health Governance* (Malden, MA: Polity Press, 2012); David P. Fidler, "Influenza Virus Samples, International Law, and Global Health Diplomacy," *Emerging Infectious Diseases* 14, no. 1 (January 2008): 88–94, https://doi.org/10.3201/eid1401.070700.

5. Nicholas Evans, *The Ethics of Neuroscience and National Security* (New York: Routledge, 2022).

6. Norman Daniels, *Just Health: Meeting Health Needs Fairly* (Cambridge: Cambridge University Press 2007).

7. Victoria Sutton, "Biodefense: Who's in Charge?," *Health Matrix: Journal of Law-Medicine* 13, no. 1 (Winter 2003): 117; Stefan Elbe, *Pandemics, Pills, and Politics: Governing Global Health Security* (Baltimore, MD: Johns Hopkins University Press, 2018); Colin McInnes and Kelley Lee, "Health, Security and Foreign Policy," *Review of International Studies* 32, no. 1 (January 2006): 5–23, https://doi.org/10.1017/S0260210506006905.

8. Peter Burnham, "Depoliticisation: Economic Crisis and Political Management," in *Tracing the Political: Depoliticisation, Governance and the State*, ed. Matt Flinders (Bristol, UK: Policy Press, 2015), 79–94.

9. Charles F. Howlett, "Studying America's Struggle against War: An Historical Perspective," *The History Teacher* 36, no. 3 (May 2003): 297–330; Joel Lefkowitz, "Movement Outcomes and Movement Decline: The Vietnam War and the Antiwar Movement," *New Political Science* 27, no. 1 (March 1, 2005): 1–22, https://doi.org/10.1080/07393140500030766; David S. Meyer, "Protest Cycles and Political Process: American Peace Movements in the Nuclear Age," *Political Research Quarterly* 46, no. 3 (September 1, 1993): 451–479, https://doi.org/10.1177/106591299304600302; Roger A. Coate, "Civil Society as a Force for Peace," *International Journal of Peace Studies* 9, no. 2 (2004): 57–86.

10. James I. Charlton, *Nothing About Us Without Us: Disability Oppression and Empowerment* (Berkeley: University of California Press, 2000), 3.

11. David France, *How to Survive a Plague: The Inside Story of How Citizens and Science Tamed AIDS.* (New York: Knopf, 2016), 413–414.

12. Thomas Hobbes, *Leviathan*, chapter XIII.

13. Jonathan Herington, "The Concept of Security, Liberty, Fear and the State," in *Security: Dialogue Across Disciplines*, ed. Philippe Bourbeau (Cambridge: Cambridge University Press, 2015), 22–44.

14. E.g., Selgelid, "A Moderate Pluralist Approach to Public Health Policy and Ethics," *Public Health Ethics* 2, no. 2 (August 2009): 195–205.

15. Robert Nozick, *Anarchy, State, and Utopia* (New York: Basic Books, 1974). For a brief overview of the central argument Nozick sets out, see Peter Vallentyne, "Robert Nozick, Anarchy, State and Utopia," in *The Twentieth Century: Quine and After* (Vol. 5 of *Central Works of Philosophy*), ed. John Shand (Stocksfield, UK: Acumen Publishing, 2006) 86–103.

16. Michael Davis, "Nozick's Argument for the Legitimacy of the Welfare State," *Ethics* 97, no. 3 (April 1987): 576–594.

17. Allen Buchanan has provided a partial reconstruction of a right to a decent minimum of healthcare based on just this. See. A. E. Buchanan, "The Right to a Decent Minimum of Health Care," *Philosophy & Public Affairs* 13, no. 1 (1984): 67.

18. We can broadly distinguish between contractualist theories that provide an account of what I can pursue based on what I can argue to others with their own interest, and contractarian theories that concern what I can pursue in bargaining with other self-interested parties. See, e.g., Michael Millar, "Constraining the Use of Antibiotics: Applying Scanlon's Contractualism," *Journal of Medical Ethics* 38, no. 8 (August 1, 2012): 465–469, https://doi.org/10.1136/medethics-2011-100256; Rahul Kumar, "Risking and Wronging," *Philosophy & Public Affairs* 43, no. 1 (2015): 27–51, https://doi.org/10.1111/papa.12042; Madison Powers et al., *Social Justice: The Moral Foundations of Public Health and Health Policy* (Oxford: Oxford University Press, 2006); Cynthia M. Jones, "The Moral Problem of Health Disparities," *American Journal of Public Health* 100, Suppl. 1 (April 2010): S47–51, https://doi.org/10.2105/AJPH.2009.171181.

19. Rawls, *A Theory of Justice* (Cambridge, MA: Harvard University Press, 1971), §24; Rawls, *Justice as Fairness: A Restatement* (Cambridge, MA: Belknap Press, 2001), 15–18.

20. Rawls, *Justice as Fairness*, §6.

21. Rawls, *Justice as Fairness*, §13.

22. Charles W. Mills, *Black Rights/White Wrongs: The Critique of Racial Liberalism* (Oxford: Oxford University Press, 2017).

23. Susan Moller Okin, *Justice, Gender, and the Family*, 3rd ed. (New York: Basic Books, 1991).

24. Norman Daniels, *Just Health: Meeting Health Needs Fairly* (Cambridge: Cambridge University Press, 2007).

25. Daniels, *Just Health*, 28–31.

26. A. E. Buchanan, "The Right to a Decent Minimum of Health Care," *Philosophy & Public Affairs* 13, no. 1 (1984): 60–61.

27. Rawls, *Justice as Fairness*, 177.

28. For a concrete example of this in the context of the Syrian Civil War, see, e.g., Nicholas Greig Evans and Mohamed A. Sekkarie, "Allocating Scarce Medical Resources during Armed Conflict: Ethical Issues," *Disaster and Military Medicine* 3, no. 1 (2017): 5, https://doi.org/10.1186/s40696-017-0033-z. For arguments applying Rawls to public health specifically, see, e.g., Selgelid, "A Moderate Pluralist Approach."

29. Piers Millett and Andrew Snyder-Beattie, "Human Agency and Global Catastrophic Biorisks," *Health Security* 15, no. 4 (August 2017): 335–336, https://doi.org/10.1089/hs.2017.0044.

30. Buchanan, "The Right to a Decent Minimum of Health Care," 60.

31. James Griffin, *Well-Being: Its Meaning, Measurement and Moral Importance* (Oxford: Oxford University Press, 1988), 42–45.

32. E.g., Christopher Boorse, "On the Distinction between Disease and Illness," *Philosophy and Public Affairs* 5, no. 1 (1975): 49–68.

33. See Owen Cotton-Barratt and Nick Bostrom, "Existential Risk and Existential Hope: Definitions," Technical Report (Oxford: Future of Humanity Institute, 2015).

34. Nick Bostrom, *Superintelligence* (Oxford: Oxford University Press, 2014).

35. John Stuart Mill, *On Liberty* (Mineola, NY: Dover Publications, 2012), 8.

36. Mill, *On Liberty*, 9.

37. See, e.g., Joel Feinberg, *Harm to Others*, reprint ed. (New York, NY: Oxford University Press, 1987). While Feinberg picks up directly from Mill, I think it's probably a mistake to consider Feinberg a utilitarian—at least, in the same way as say Peter Singer. Indeed, his at times contractarian and dignitarian leanings seem to come to the fore. See, e.g., J. Angelo Corlett, "The Philosophy of Joel Feinberg," *Journal of Ethics* 10, no. 1/2 (2006): 131–132.

38. Interestingly, though not critically to this work, the US Libertarian Party's 2016 manifesto includes a nod to the harm principle: "Criminal laws should be limited in their application to violations of the rights of others through force or fraud, *or to deliberate actions that place others involuntarily at significant risk of harm*" (emphasis added).

39. Michael Moehler, *Minimal Morality: A Multilevel Social Contract Theory* (Oxford: Oxford University Press, 2018), 6–7.

40. Jennifer Flynn, "Theory and Bioethics," in *The Stanford Encyclopedia of Philosophy*, ed. Edward N. Zalta (Palo Alto, CA: Stanford University Press, 2020), https://plato.stanford.edu/archives/win2020/entriesheory-bioethics/.

41. Tom L. Beauchamp and James F. Childress, *Principles of Biomedical Ethics* (New York: Oxford University Press, 2012), ch. 2.

42. Jonathan D. Moreno, "Bioethics Is a Naturalism," in *Pramgatic Bioethics*, ed. Glenn McGee (Cambridge, MA: MIT Press, 1999), 8. See also Jonathan D. Moreno, *Deciding Together: Bioethics and Moral Consensus* (New York: Oxford University Press, 1995).

It is worth noting—as part of the history of ideas aspect of this project—that the pragmatist tradition in bioethics has been largely silent since the departure of one of its greatest proponents, Glenn McGee. McGee's departure is controversial and there remain questions about his actions, and his relation to the larger norms of the field. See Brendan Borrell, "An Unethical Ethicist?," *Scientific American*, 2006, https://www.scientificamerican.com/article/glenn-mcgee/; Ivan Oransky, "Updated: Slate Retracts Story on Glenn McGee and Celltex Following Lawsuit Threats, as McGee Resigns from Company," *Retraction Watch* (blog), March 1, 2012, https://retractionwatch.com/2012/03/01/slate-retracts-story-on-glenn-mcgee-and-celltex-as-mcgee-resigns-from-company/; Alice Domurat Dreger, *Galileo's Middle Finger: Heretics, Activists, and the Search for Justice in Science* (New York: Penguin Press, 2015).

43. Selgelid, "A Moderate Pluralist Approach."

44. Moehler, *Minimal Morality*.

45. Michael Moehler, "The Rawls–Harsanyi Dispute: A Moral Point of View," *Pacific Philosophical Quarterly* 99, no. 1 (2018): 82–99, https://doi.org/10.1111/papq.12140.

46. Moehler, *Minimal Morality*, 114.

47. US Centers for Disease Control and Prevention, "Burden of Influenza," April 17, 2020, https://www.cdc.gov/flu/about/burden/index.html.

48. Luciana Borio, "21st Century Pandemic, Prehistoric Clinical Trials," *BioCentury*, June 26, 2020, https://www.biocentury.com/article/305565/21st-century-pandemic -prehistoric-clinical-trials?editionId=ckbx19vog0y5v01678lszox0w.

49. Kai Kupferschmidt, "One U.K. Trial Is Transforming COVID-19 Treatment: Why Haven't Others Delivered More Results?" *Science*, July 2, 2020, https://doi.org/10 .1126/science.abd6417.

50. Michael Moehler, "In Defense of a Democratic Productivist Welfare State," *European Journal of Philosophy* 25, no. 2 (June 2017): 416–439, https://doi.org/10.1111/ejop .12157.

51. Wayan C. W. S. Putri et al., "Economic Burden of Seasonal Influenza in the United States," *Vaccine* 36, no. 27 (June 22, 2018): 3960–3966, https://doi.org/10.1016/j.vaccine .2018.05.057.

52. All data are drawn from public website data at cdc.gov.

53. R. Crawford, "Healthism and the Medicalization of Everyday Life," *International Journal of Health Services: Planning, Administration, Evaluation* 10, no. 3 (1980): 365– 388, https://doi.org/10.2190/3H2H-3XJN-3KAY-G9NY.

54. See Hereth et al., "Long COVID: Brave New World."

55. Zackary D. Berger et al., "Covid-19: Control Measures Must Be Equitable and Inclusive," *BMJ*, March 20, 2020, m1141.

56. Emily Stewart, "Anti-Maskers Explain Themselves," Vox, August 7, 2020, https://www.vox.com/the-goods/2020/8/7/21357400/anti-mask-protest-rallies -donald-trump-covid-19.

57. Moehler, *Minimal Morality*, 99–100.

Chapter 6

1. David N. Durrheim, Laurence O. Gostin, and Keymanthri Moodley, "When Does a Major Outbreak Become a Public Health Emergency of International Concern?,"

The Lancet Infectious Diseases 20, no. 8 (August 1, 2020): 887–889, https://doi.org/10 .1016/S1473-3099(20)30401-1.

2. Michael Levenson, "Scale of China's Wuhan Shutdown Is Believed to Be Without Precedent," *New York Times*, January 23, 2020, sec. World, https://www.nytimes .com/2020/01/22/world/asia/coronavirus-quarantines-history.html.

3. Roojin Habibi et al., "Do Not Violate the International Health Regulations during the COVID-19 Outbreak," *The Lancet* 395, no. 10225 (February 29, 2020): 664–666, https://doi.org/10.1016/S0140-6736(20)30373-1.

4. *International Health Regulations*, Annex 2.

5. Mark Eccleston-Turner and Adam Kamradt-Scott, "Transparency in IHR Emergency Committee Decision Making: The Case for Reform," *BMJ Global Health* 4, no. 2 (April 1, 2019): e001618, https://doi.org/10.1136/bmjgh-2019-001618.

6. Stafford Act, 1.

7. PHSA, §319.

8. MSEHPA, §104 (m).

9. Indiana Code, §10-14-3. See Rebecca Haffajee, Wendy E. Parmet, and Michelle M. Mello, "What Is a Public Health 'Emergency'?," *New England Journal of Medicine* 371, no. 11 (September 11, 2014): 986–988, https://doi.org/10.1056/NEJMp1406167.

10. Adam Gaber, "Liberia Adopts Yale Capstone Recommendations for Medical Education Reform," YaleNews, April 30, 2018, https://news.yale.edu/2018/04/30/liberia -adopts-yale-capstone-recommendations-medical-education-reform.

11. David K. Evans, Markus Goldstein, and Anna Popova, "Health-Care Worker Mortality and the Legacy of the Ebola Epidemic," *The Lancet Global Health* 3, no. 8 (August 2015): e439–440, https://doi.org/10.1016/S2214-109X(15)00065-0.

12. Kelly Hills, "Rejecting Quarantine," in *Ebola's Message*, ed. Nicholas Greig Evans, Tara C. Smith, and Maimuna S. Majumder (Cambridge, MA: MIT Press, 2016), 217–231.

13. Nicholas G. Evans, "Covid-19: The Ethics of Clinical Research in Quarantine," *BMJ* 369 (May 29, 2020), https://doi.org/10.1136/bmj.m2060.

14. See G. M. Reichert, "Jus ad bellum," in *War*, ed. Larry May (Cambridge: Cambridge University Press, 2008), 13–14.

15. NBC Connecticut, "Governor Declares Cautionary Public Health Emergency Over Ebola," *NBC Connecticut*, October 7, 2014, https://www.nbcconnecticut.com/news /local/governor-declares-state-of-emergency-over-ebola-as-a-precaution/59231/.

16. Sheri Fink, "Connecticut Faces Lawsuit Over Ebola Quarantine Policies (Published 2016)," *New York Times*, February 7, 2016, sec. New York, https://www.nytimes.com

/2016/02/08/nyregion/connecticut-faces-lawsuit-over-ebola-quarantine-policies
.html.

17. Greg Allen, "From Alaska to Florida, States Respond to Opioid Crisis with Emergency Declarations," NPR.org, accessed December 30, 2020, https://www.npr.org/sections/health-shots/2017/08/11/542836709/from-alaska-to-florida-states-respond-to-opioid-crisis-with-emergency-declaratio.

18. Rebecca Haffajee, Wendy E. Parmet, and Michelle M. Mello, "What Is a Public Health 'Emergency'?," *New England Journal of Medicine* 371, no. 11 (September 11, 2014): 986–988, https://doi.org/10.1056/NEJMp1406167.

19. Thomas Hurka, "Proportionality and Necessity," in *War*, ed. Larry May (Cambridge: Cambridge University Press, 2008), 127–144.

20. Ruth Chang, *Incommensurability, Incomparability, and Practical Reason* (Cambridge, MA: Harvard University Press, 1997).

21. University of Auckland et al., "COVID-19 among Indigenous Communities: Case Studies on Indigenous Nursing Responses in Australia, Canada, New Zealand, and the United States," *Nursing Praxis Aotearoa New Zealand*, December 2021, 71–83, https://doi.org/10.36951/27034542.2021.037; Nikki Moodie et al., "Roadmap to Recovery: Reporting on a Research Taskforce Supporting Indigenous Responses to COVID-19 in Australia," *Australian Journal of Social Issues* 56, no. 1 (2021): 4–16, https://doi.org/10.1002/ajs4.133; Gwendolyn Saul, Kerry F. Thompson, and Lisa Hardy, "Tribes Mount Organized Responses to COVID-19, in Contrast to State and Federal Governments," The Conversation, December 2, 2020, http://theconversation.com/tribes-mount-organized-responses-to-covid-19-in-contrast-to-state-and-federal-governments-150627.

22. Michael Walzer, *Just and Unjust Wars: A Moral Argument with Historical Illustrations*, 4th ed. (New York: Basic Books, 2006), preface, esp. xiv–xv; cf. C. A. J. Coady, *Morality and Political Violence* (Cambridge: Cambridge University Press, 2007).

23. Shannon Brandt Ford, "Jus Ad Vim and the Just Use of Lethal Force Short of War," in *Routledge Handbook of Ethics and War: Just War Theory in the 21st Century*, ed. Fritz Allhoff, Nicholas Evans, and Adam Henschke (London: Routledge, 2013), 63–75; Megan Braun and Daniel R. Brunstetter, "Rethinking the Criterion for Assessing CIA-Targeted Killings: Drones, Proportionality and Jus Ad Vim," *Journal of Military Ethics* 12, no. 4 (December 2013): 304–324, https://doi.org/10.1080/15027570.2013.869390.

24. Kelsey D. Atherton, "Trump Inherited the Drone War but Ditched Accountability," *Foreign Policy* (blog), May 22, 2020, https://foreignpolicy.com/2020/05/22/obama-drones-trump-killings-count/.

25. Daniel B. Kelly, "The Public Use Requirement in Eminent Domain Law: A Rationale Based on Secret Purchases and Private Influence," *Cornell Law Journal* 92 (2006): 56.

26. Julian Savulescu, "Good Reasons to Vaccinate: Mandatory or Payment for Risk?," *Journal of Medical Ethics*, November 9, 2020, https://doi.org/10.1136/medethics-2020 -106821; cf. Lawrence O. Gostin, Daniel A. Salmon, and Heidi J. Larson, "Mandating COVID-19 Vaccines," *JAMA*, December 29, 2020, https://doi.org/10.1001/jama.2020 .26553.

27. Katie Attwell et al., "Financial Interventions to Increase Vaccine Coverage," *Pediatrics* 146, no. 6 (December 1, 2020), https://doi.org/10.1542/peds.2020-0724; though cf. Joshua T. B. Williams and Simon J. Hambidge, "Effectiveness and Equity of Australian Vaccine Mandates," *Pediatrics* 146, no. 6 (December 1, 2020), https://doi.org/10 .1542/peds.2020-024703.

28. Efthimios Parasidis, "Public Health Law and Institutional Vaccine Skepticism," *Journal of Health Politics, Policy and Law* 41, no. 6 (December 1, 2016): 1137–1149, https://doi.org/10.1215/03616878-3666204.

29. For issues related to how we structure our priorities around issues of moral will, see, e.g., Regina Brown and Nicholas Greig Evans, "The Social Value of Candidate HIV Cures: Actualism versus Possibilism," *Journal of Medical Ethics*, July 2016, medethics-2015–103125, https://doi.org/10.1136/medethics-2015-103125.

30. Marcia Baron, "Self-Defense: The Imminence Requirement," in *Oxford Studies in Philosophy of Law* (Oxford: Oxford University Press, 2011); Daniel Schwartz, "Necessity Historically Considered," *Journal of Moral Philosophy* 17, no. 6 (April 13, 2020): 591–605, https://doi.org/10.1163/17455243-20203185.

Chapter 7

1. Donald A. Henderson et al., "A Plague on Your City: Observations from TOPOFF," *Clinical Infectious Diseases* 32, no. 3 (February 1, 2001): 436–445, https://doi.org/10 .1086/318513; John D. Blum, "Too Strange to Be Just Fiction: Legal Lessons from a Bioterrorist Simulation, the Case of TOPOFF 2," *Louisiana Law Review* 2, no. 64 (2000): 905–917.

2. Kelly Hills, "Rejecting Quarantine," in *Ebola's Message*, ed. Nicholas Greig Evans, Tara C. Smith, and Maimuna S. Majumder (Cambridge, MA: MIT Press, 2016), 217–231.

3. The COVID-LOCAL Analysis and Mapping of Policies lists no state-level distancing measure as "lockdown" during 2020. See https://covidamp.org/policymaps.

4. Phil Mercer, "Covid: Melbourne's Hard-Won Success after a Marathon Lockdown," *BBC News*, October 26, 2020, sec. Australia, https://www.bbc.com/news/world-australia -54654646.

5. Kun Liu et al., "Population Movement, City Closure in Wuhan, and Geographical Expansion of the COVID-19 Infection in China in January 2020," *Clinical Infectious Diseases* 71, no. 16 (November 19, 2020): 2045–2051, https://doi.org/10.1093/cid

/ciaa422; Zheming Yuan et al., "Modelling the Effects of Wuhan's Lockdown during COVID-19, China," *Bulletin of the World Health Organization* 98 (2020): 484–494, https://doi.org/10.2471/BLT.20.254045.

6. Kai Kupferschmidt and John Cohen, "China's Aggressive Measures Have Slowed the Coronavirus: They May Not Work in Other Countries," *Science Insider*, March 2, 2020, https://www.science.org/content/article/china-s-aggressive-measures-have -slowed-coronavirus-they-may-not-work-other-countries.

7. Potter, "We Are at War with COVID-19: We Need to Fight It Like a War," *Globe and Mail*, April 5, 2020. https://www.theglobeandmail.com/opinion/article-we-are -at-war-with-covid-19-we-need-to-fight-it-like-a-war/.

8. See, e.g., Seth Lazar, *Sparing Civilians* (Oxford: Oxford University Press, 2016).

9. Seth Lazar, "Morality & Law of War," in *Companion to Philosophy of Law*, ed. Andrei Marmor (New York: Routledge), 364–379.

10. See, e.g., Gerhard Øverland, "High-Fliers: Who Should bear the Risk of Humanitarian Intervention?" in *New Wars and New Soldiers: Military Ethics in the Contemporary World*, ed. Paolo Tripodi and Jessica Wolfendale (London: Ashgate, 2012).

11. Seth Lazar, *Sparing Civilians* (Oxford: Oxford University Press, 2016).

12. May, *Contingent Pacifism: Revisiting Just War Theory* (Cambridge: Cambridge University Press, 2015), 160.

13. May, *Contingent Pacifism*, 161–163.

14. International Court of Justice, "Legality of the Threat of Nuclear Weapons," § 24, 17.

15. Famously, Jeff McMahan, "Innocence, Self-Defense and Killing in War," *Journal of Political Philosophy* 2, no. 3 (September 1994): 193–221; J. McMahan, *The Ethics of Killing: Problems at the Margins of Life* (Oxford: Oxford University Press, 2002); J. McMahan, "Who Is Morally Liable to Be Killed in War," *Analysis* 71, no. 3 (July 2011): 544–559, https://doi.org/10.1093/analys/anr072.

16. Sara Jensen Carr. "The Topography of Wellness: Mechanisms, Metrics, and Models of Health in the Urban Landscape" (PhD dissertation, University of California–Berkeley, 2014), https://escholarship.org/uc/item/8cg2t860.

17. Margaret Campbell, "What Tuberculosis Did for Modernism: The Influence of a Curative Environment on Modernist Design and Architecture," *Medical History* 49, no. 4 (October 1, 2005): 463–488.

18. CDC, "Quarantine & Isolation," Centers for Disease Control and Prevention, January 27, 2022, https://www.cdc.gov/coronavirus/2019-ncov/your-health/quarantine -isolation.html. For a description of the risks and conflation of the two, see Hills, "Rejecting Quarantine."

19. Zackary D. Berger, Nicholas G. Evans, Alexandra L. Phelan, and Ross D. Silverman, "Covid-19: Control Measures Must Be Equitable and Inclusive," *BMJ* 368 (March 20, 2020), https://doi.org/10.1136/bmj.m1141.

20. WHO Newsroom, "Ciclovías Temporales, Bogotá, Colombia," accessed January 26, 2021, https://www.who.int/news-room/feature-stories/detail/ciclovías-temporales-bogotá-colombia.

21. See, e.g., COVID-19 LOCAL for an overview and detail of measures. The comparative effectiveness of these is beyond the scope, unfortunately, of this work.

22. Matthew K. Wynia, "Ethics and Public Health Emergencies: Restrictions on Liberty," *American Journal of Bioethics: AJOB* 7, no. 2 (February 2007): 1–5, https://doi.org/10.1080/15265160701577603; Hills, "Rejecting Quarantine"; Lawrence O. Gostin et al., "The Model State Emergency Health Powers Act: Planning for and Response to Bioterrorism and Naturally Occurring Infectious Diseases," *JAMA* 288, no. 5 (August 7, 2002): 622–628, https://doi.org/10.1001/jama.288.5.622; Lawrence O. Gostin, "When Terrorism Threatens Health: How Far Are Limitations on Human Rights Justified," *Journal of Law, Medicine & Ethics* 31, no. 4 (December 1, 2003): 524–528, https://doi.org/10.1111/j.1748-720X.2003.tb00120.x; Lindsay F. Wiley, "Democratizing the Law of Social Distancing," SSRN Scholarly Paper (Rochester, NY: Social Science Research Network, June 24, 2020), https://doi.org/10.2139/ssrn.3634997; W. E. Parmet, "Quarantine Redux: Bioterrorism, AIDS and the Curtailment of Individual Liberty in the Name of Public Health," *Health Matrix*, 2003, http://heinonline.org/hol-cgi-bin/get_pdf.cgi?handle=hein.journals/hmax13&section=10; Griffin Trotter, *The Ethics of Coercion in Mass Casualty Medicine* (Baltimore, MD: Johns Hopkins University Press, 2007); Nicholas G. Evans, "Covid-19: The Ethics of Clinical Research in Quarantine," *BMJ* 369 (May 29, 2020), https://doi.org/10.1136/bmj.m2060.

23. N. Ferguson, D. Laydon, G. Nedjati Gilani, N. Imai, K. Ainslie, M. Baguelin, S. Bhatia, et al., "Report 9: Impact of Non-Pharmaceutical Interventions (NPIs) to Reduce COVID19 Mortality and Healthcare Demand" (London: Imperial College, March 16, 2020), https://doi.org/10.25561/77482; Matteo Chinazzi, Jessica T. Davis, Marco Ajelli, Corrado Gioannini, Maria Litvinova, Stefano Merler, Ana Pastore y Piontti, et al., "The Effect of Travel Restrictions on the Spread of the 2019 Novel Coronavirus (COVID-19) Outbreak," *Science* 368, no. 6489 (April 24, 2020): 395–400, https://doi.org/10.1126/science.aba9757.

24. Cameron McWhirter and Valier Bauerlein, "Georgia Reopens but Many Businesses Stay Closed, People Stay Home," *Wall Street Journal*, April 24, 2020, sec. US, https://www.wsj.com/articles/georgia-reopens-but-many-businesses-stay-closed-people-stay-home-11587754211.

25. James F. Childress and Ruth Gaare Bernheim, "Beyond the Liberal and Communitarian Impasse: A Framework and Vision for Public Health," *Florida Law Review* 55, no. 5 (2003): 1191–1291.

26. See, e.g., Wynia, "Ethics and Public Health Emergencies."

27. Philip Pettit, "Consequentialism and Respect for Persons," *Ethics* 100, no. 1 (October 1989): 116–126, https://doi.org/10.2307/2381149?ref=search-gateway:f6dfa036817 7ed4f28320943db714f48; Philip Pettit, "The Consequentialist Can Recognise Rights," *The Philosophical Quarterly* 38, no. 150 (January 1988): 42–55, https://doi.org/10.2307 /2220266; Phillip Pettit, *Republicanism: A Theory of Freedom and Government*, (Oxford: Oxford University Press, 1997).

28. Frank Shechtman, "Routine Medical Care May Break Down, and Covid-19 Is Behind It," *New York Times*, March 23, 2020, sec. Opinion, https://www.nytimes .com/2020/03/23/opinion/doctors-coronavirus-patients.html.

29. Robert E. Goodin, *Protecting the Vulnerable* (Chicago: University of Chicago Press, 1984).

30. Caroline Bettinger-Lopez, and Alexandra Bro, "A Double Pandemic: Domestic Violence in the Age of COVID-19," Council on Foreign Relations, May 13, 2020, https://www.cfr.org/in-brief/double-pandemic-domestic-violence-age-covid-19.

31. Michael Grabell and Bernice Yeung, "Meatpacking Companies Dismissed Years of Warnings but Now Say Nobody Could Have Prepared for COVID-19," ProPublica, accessed January 26, 2021, https://www.propublica.org/article/meatpacking-companies -dismissed-years-of-warnings-but-now-say-nobody-could-have-prepared-for-covid-19 ?token=8x14roDzBQ5p8Y0hCArCtdwGWCNrGooB; Michelle A. Waltenburg, "Update: COVID-19 Among Workers in Meat and Poultry Processing Facilities—United States, April–May 2020," *MMWR. Morbidity and Mortality Weekly Report* 69 (2020), https://doi .org/10.15585/mmwr.mm6927e2.

32. Linda Moy, Hildegard K. Toth, Mary S. Newell, Donna Plecha, Jessica W. T. Leung, and Jennifer A. Harvey, "Response to COVID-19 in Breast Imaging," *Journal of Breast Imaging*, April 1, 2020, https://doi.org/10.1093/jbi/wbaa025.

33. J. Michael McGinnis and William H. Foege, "Actual Causes of Death in the United States," *JAMA* 270, no. 18 (November 10, 1993): 2207–2212, https://doi.org /10.1001/jama.1993.03510180077038.

34. See, e.g., Arline T. Geronimus et al., "'Weathering' and Age Patterns of Allostatic Load Scores among Blacks and Whites in the United States," *American Journal of Public Health* 96, no. 5 (May 2006): 826–833, https://doi.org/10.2105/AJPH.2004.060749.

35. Berger et al., "Covid-19."

36. Timothy Allen and Michael J. Selgelid, "Necessity and Least Infringement Conditions in Public Health Ethics," *Medicine, Health Care and Philosophy* 20 (April 2017): 525–535, https://doi.org/10.1007/s11019-017-9775-0.

37. Seth Lazar, *Sparing Civilians*, 81–83.

38. *Sparing Civilians*, 84–85.

39. Nicholas Greig Evans and Thomas Inglesby, "Biosecurity and Public Health Ethics Issues Raised by Biological Threats," in *The Oxford Handbook of Public Health Ethics*, ed. Anna C. Mastroianni, Jeffrey P. Kahn, and Nancy E. Kass (Oxford: Oxford University Press, 2019), 773–785.

40. Myah Ward, "We're Not Ready for the Next Pandemic," POLITICO, accessed February 4, 2022, https://politi.co/2Y1llB7; Bryan Walsh, "The World Is Not Ready for the Next Pandemic," *Time*, May 4, 2017, https://time.com/magazine/us/4766607 /may-15th-2017-vol-189-no-18-u-s/; Andrew C. Heinrich and Saad B. Omer, "The World Isn't Ready for the Next Outbreak," September 23, 2021, https://www .foreignaffairs.com/articles/world/2021-09-06/world-isnt-ready-next-outbreak; Maggie Fox, "The World Is Unprepared for the next Pandemic, Study Finds," CNN, accessed February 4, 2022, https://www.cnn.com/2021/12/08/health/world -unprepared-pandemic-report/index.html; Andy Plump, "Luck Is Not a Strategy: The World Needs to Start Preparing Now for the Next Pandemic," *STAT* (blog), May 18, 2021, https://www.statnews.com/2021/05/18/luck-is-not-a-strategy-the-world-needs -to-start-preparing-now-for-the-next-pandemic/.

41. Sun Tzu, *The Art of War* (Courier Corporation, 2012), §1.

42. White House, "Opening Up America Again," The White House, 2020, https://www .whitehouse.gov/openingamerica/; Scott Gottlieb, Caitlin Rivers, Mark B. McClellan, Lauren Silvis, and Crystal Watson, "National Coronavirus Response" (Washington DC: American Enterprise Institute, March 28, 2020); Zeke Emanuel, T. Neera, Topher Spiro, Adam Conner, Kevin DeGood, Erin Simpson, Nicole Rapfogel, and Maura Calsyn, "A National and State Plan to End the Coronavirus Crisis," Center for American Prog- ress, April 3, 2020, https://www.americanprogress.org/issues/healthcare/news/2020 /04/03/482613/national-state-plan-end-coronavirus-crisis/; Vital Strategies, "Box It In: Rapid Public Health Action Can Box in COVID-19 and Reopen Society," 2020, https://preventepidemics.org/wp-content/uploads/2020/04/BoxItInBriefingDoc.pdf; Danielle Allen, Sharon Block, Joshua Cohen, Peter Eckersley, M. Eifler, Lawrence Gostin, Darshan Goux, et al., "Roadmap to Pandemic Resilience," 2020, https:// ethics.harvard.edu/covid-roadmap.

43. Centers for Disease Control and Prevention, "SARS, CDC Guidance Supplement D: Community Containment Measures, Including Non-Hospital Isolation and Quar- antine," February 8, 2019, https://www.cdc.gov/sars/guidance/d-quarantine/comm unity.html.

44. Vital Strategies, "Box It In."

45. Allen et al., "Roadmap to Pandemic Resilience."

46. Ferguson et al., "Report 9."

47. Evans and Inglesby, "Biosecurity and Public Health Ethics Issues."

48. Katherine A. Auger et al., "Association Between Statewide School Closure and COVID-19 Incidence and Mortality in the US," *JAMA*, July 29, 2020, https://doi.org/10.1001/jama.2020.14348; Jan M. Brauner et al., "Inferring the Effectiveness of Government Interventions against COVID-19," *Science*, December 15, 2020, https://doi.org/10.1126/science.abd9338; An Pan et al., "Association of Public Health Interventions with the Epidemiology of the COVID-19 Outbreak in Wuhan, China," *JAMA*, April 10, 2020, https://doi.org/10.1001/jama.2020.6130; Bryan Wilder et al., "Modeling Between-Population Variation in COVID-19 Dynamics in Hubei, Lombardy, and New York City," *Proceedings of the National Academy of Sciences*, September 24, 2020, https://doi.org/10.1073/pnas.2010651117.

49. Allen and Selgelid, "Necessity and Least Infringement Conditions."

50. May, *Contingent Pacifism*.

51. Heejin Kim, Sohee Kim, and Claire Che, "Virus Testing Blitz Appears to Keep Korea Death Rate Low," *Bloomberg.Com*, March 4, 2020, https://www.bloomberg.com/news/articles/2020-03-04/south-korea-tests-hundreds-of-thousands-to-fight-virus-outbreak; Solomon Hsiang et al., "The Effect of Large-Scale Anti-Contagion Policies on the COVID-19 Pandemic," *Nature*, June 8, 2020, 1–9, https://doi.org/10.1038/s41586-020-2404-8; June-Ho Kim et al., "Emerging COVID-19 Success Story: South Korea Learned the Lessons of MERS," Our World in Data, 2021, https://ourworldindata.org/covid-exemplar-south-korea; Derek Thompson, "What's Behind South Korea's COVID-19 Exceptionalism?," *The Atlantic*, May 6, 2020, https://www.theatlantic.com/ideas/archive/2020/05/whats-south-koreas-secret/611215/; Wudan Yan and Anne Babe, "What Should the U.S. Learn from South Korea's Covid-19 Success?," Undark Magazine, October 5, 2020, https://undark.org/2020/10/05/south-korea-covid-19-success/.

52. See, e.g., Evans, "Covid-19."

Chapter 8

1. David von Drehle, "The Ebola Fighters," *Time*, December 10, 2014, https://time.com/time-person-of-the-year-ebola-fighters/.

2. David K. Evans, Markus Goldstein, and Anna Popova, "Health-Care Worker Mortality and the Legacy of the Ebola Epidemic," *The Lancet Global Health* 3, no. 8 (August 2015): e439–440, https://doi.org/10.1016/S2214-109X(15)00065-0.

3. Julia Lynch et al., "Ignoring Nurses: Media Coverage during the COVID-19 Pandemic," *Annals of the American Thoracic Society*, February 12, 2021, https://doi.org/10.1513/AnnalsATS.202010-1293PS.

4. Nicholas Greig Evans, "Balancing the Duty to Treat Patients with Ebola Virus Disease with the Risks to Dialysis Personnel," *Clinical Journal of the American Society*

of Nephrology 10, no. 12 (August 2015): CJN.03730415–2267, https://doi.org/10.2215 /CJN.03730415.

5. National Conference of State Legislatures, "COVID-19: Essential Workers in the States," January 11, 2021, https://www.ncsl.org/research/labor-and-employment/covid -19-essential-workers-in-the-states.aspx.

6. Aaron Mehta, "Pentagon Declares Defense Contractors 'Critical Infrastructure,' Must Continue Work," Defense News, March 20, 2020, https://www.defensenews.com /pentagon/2020/03/20/pentagon-declares-defense-contractors-critical-infrastructure -must-continue-work/.

7. Nick Brown and Christina Cook, "In Fight for Masks, Hospital Janitors Some-times Come Last," *Reuters,* April 6, 2020, https://www.reuters.com/article/us-health -coronavirus-housekeepers/in-fight-for-masks-hospital-janitors-sometimes-come-last -idUSKBN21O2JF.

8. Norman Daniels, "Duty to Treat or Right to Refuse?," *The Hastings Center Report* 21, no. 2 (1991): 36, https://doi.org/10.2307/3562338; Torben K. Becker et al., "Ethical Challenges in Emergency Medical Services: Controversies and Recommendations," *Prehospital and Disaster Medicine* 28, no. 5 (October 2013): 488–497, https://doi.org/10 .1017/S1049023X13008728.

9. Nicholas Greig Evans, "Balancing the Duty to Treat Patients with Ebola Virus Disease with the Risks to Dialysis Personnel," *Clinical Journal of the American Society of Nephrology* 10, no. 12 (August 2015): CJN.03730415–2267, https://doi.org/10.2215 /CJN.03730415.

10. Leigh Turner, "Bioethics, Public Health, and Firearm-Related Violence: Missing Links between Bioethics and Public Health," *Journal of Law, Medicine & Ethics* 25, no. 1 (March 1997): 42–48, https://doi.org/10.1111/j.1748-720X.1997.tb01395.x.

11. Patrick Mileham, "Unlimited Liability and the Military Covenant," *Journal of Military Ethics* 9, no. 1 (March 1, 2010): 23–40, https://doi.org/10.1080/15027570903 353836.

12. See Larry May, *Contingent Pacifism: Revisiting Just War Theory* (Cambridge: Cambridge University Press, 2015), ch. 5.

13. Alfred, Lord Tennyson, "The Charge of the Light Brigade" in *Maud, and Other Poems* (1850).

14. Donald A. Henderson et al., "A Plague on Your City: Observations from TOPOFF," *Clinical Infectious Diseases* 32, no. 3 (February 1, 2001): 436–445, https://doi.org/10 .1086/318513.

15. Sean McDonald, "Ebola: A Big Data Disaster," accessed December 31, 2020, https://www.academia.edu/21348760/Ebola_A_Big_Data_Disaster.

16. McDonald, "Ebola."

17. See, e.g., Seumas Miller, *The Moral Foundations of Social Institutions, A Philosophical Study* (Cambridge: Cambridge University Press, 2010).

18. "Dying in a Leadership Vacuum," editorial, *New England Journal of Medicine* 383, no. 15 (October 8, 2020): 1479–1480, https://doi.org/10.1056/NEJMe2029812.

19 H. Holden Thorp, "It Ain't Over 'til It's Over," *Science* 376, no. 6594 (May 13, 2022): 675–675, https://doi.org/10.1126/science.abq8460.

20. Not institutional leaders, strictly speaking, given my earlier moral characterization of institutions.

21. See Evans, *The Ethics of Neuroscience and National Security* (New York: Routledge, 2022), ch. 8.

22. Derek Thompson, "American Elites Still Don't Understand How COVID-19 Works," *The Atlantic*, December 11, 2020, https://www.theatlantic.com/ideas/archive/2020/12/americas-bipartisan-covid-19-illiteracy/617368/.

23. Rachel Martin, "Trump Tells Woodward He Deliberately Downplayed Coronavirus Threat," NPR, September 10, 2020, sec. Politics, https://www.npr.org/2020/09/10/911368698/trump-tells-woodward-he-deliberately-downplayed-coronavirus-threat.

24. Lenny Bernstein and Lena H. Sun, "CDC Director Allegedly Ordered Deletion of Email Showing Effort to Interfere with Coronavirus Guidance, Lawmaker Says," *Washington Post*, accessed December 31, 2020, https://www.washingtonpost.com/health/covid-cdc-director-email/2020/12/10/bc72461a-3af3-11eb-9276-ae0ca72729be_story.html.

25. Mike Stobbe, *Surgeon General's Warning: How Politics Crippled the Nation's Doctor* (Oakland: University of California Press, 2014).

26. "Everyone Has an Opinion on Queensland's Border Restrictions, but Who Has the Final Say?," *ABC News*, October 14, 2020, https://www.abc.net.au/news/2020-10-15/queensland-coronavirus-borders-whos-in-charge/12753776; "Chief Health Officers Are in the Spotlight Like Never Before: Here's What Goes on behind the Scenes | School of Population Health," n.d., https://sph.med.unsw.edu.au/news/chief-health-officers-are-spotlight-never-heres-what-goes-behind-scenes.

27. "Emails Reveal Sutton's Concern about 'Wrong Cohort' Staffing Quarantine Hotels," *ABC News*, September 16, 2020, https://www.abc.net.au/news/2020-09-16/brett-sutton-victorian-coronavirus-hotel-quarantine-inquiry/12668398.

28. Lawrence O. Gostin, "Public Health, Ethics, and Human Rights: A Tribute to the Late Jonathan Mann," *Journal of Law, Medicine & Ethics* 29, no. 2 (June 1, 2001): 121–130, https://doi.org/10.1111/j.1748-720X.2001.tb00330.x.

Chapter 9

1. Brian Orend, "Jus Post Bellum," *Journal of Social Philosophy* 31, no. 1 (2000): 117–137, https://doi.org/10.1111/0047-2786.00034; Brian Orend, *The Morality of War* (Peterborough, ON: Broadview Press, 2006).

2. Gregg Gonsalves, "The Moral Danger of Declaring the Pandemic Over Too Soon," *New York Times*, February 17, 2022, https://www.nytimes.com/2022/02/17/opinion /aids-pandemic-covid.html.

3. H. Holden Thorp, "It Ain't Over 'til It's Over," *Science* 376, no. 6594 (May 13, 2022): 675–675, https://doi.org/10.1126/science.abq8460.

4. Brian Orend, "Jus Post Bellum."

5. G. Blum and D. Luban, "Unsatisfying Wars: Degrees of Risk and the Jus Ex Bello," *Ethics* 125, no. 3 (2015): 751–780, https://doi.org/10.1086/679558; D. Moellendorf, "Two Doctrines of Jus Ex Bello," *Ethics* 125, no. 3 (2015): 653–673, https://doi.org/10 .1086/679560; D. Statman, "Ending War Short of Victory? A Contractarian View of Jus Ex Bello," *Ethics* 125, no. 3 (2015): 720–750, https://doi.org/10.1086/679561.

6. Larry May, *War Crimes and Just War* (Cambridge: Cambridge University Press, 2007).

7. Robert E. Williams, "Jus Post Bellum: Justice in the Aftermath of War," in *The Future of Just War*, ed. Caron E. Gentry and Amy E. Eckert, New Critical Essays (University of Georgia Press, 2014), 167–180, https://doi.org/10.2307/j.ctt46nbn3.13.

8. James Pattison, "Jus Post Bellum and the Responsibility to Rebuild," *British Journal of Political Science* 45, no. 3 (July 2015): 635–661, https://doi.org/10.1017 /S0007123413000331.

9. Pattinson, "Jus Post Bellum," 638–639.

10. Aris Katzourakis, *Nature* 601 (2022): 485, https://doi.org/10.1038/d41586-022 -00155-x.

11 Martha Lincoln and Lorenzo Servitje, "Biden's 'New Normal' on COVID Is Neither Normal nor New," *Salon* June 26, 2022, https://www.salon.com/2022/06/26 /biden-new-normal/.

12. Smriti Mallapaty, "COVID Is Spreading in Deer: What Does That Mean for the Pandemic?" *Nature* 604, no. 7907 (April 28, 2022): 612–615, https://doi.org/10.1038 /d41586-022-01112-4.

13. Daniel Schwartz, "Necessity Historically Considered," *Journal of Moral Philosophy* 17, no. 6 (April 13, 2020): 591–605, https://doi.org/10.1163/17455243-20203185.

14. Abigail Cartus and Justin Feldman, "Motivated Reasoning: Emily Oster's COVID Narratives and the Attack on Public Education," *Protean Magazine,* March 22, 2022,

https://proteanmag.com/2022/03/22/motivated-reasoning-emily-osters-covid
-narratives-and-the-attack-on-public-education/.

Chapter 10

1. Mike Stobbe, *Surgeon General's Warning: How Politics Crippled the Nation's Doctor* (Oakland: University of California Press, 2014), 137–145.

2. Clifford Marks, "Inside the American Medical Association's Fight Over Single-Payer Health Care," *New Yorker*, July 11, 2022, https://www.newyorker.com/science /annals-of-medicine/the-fight-within-the-american-medical-association.

3. Senate Committee on Health, Education, Labor, and Pensions, "Murray and Burr Release Discussion Draft of Bipartisan Pandemic and Public Health Preparedness and Response Bill," accessed February 5, 2022, https://www.help.senate.gov/chair /newsroom/press/murray-and-burr-release-discussion-draft-of-bipartisan-pandemic -and-public-health-preparedness-and-response-bill.

4. Nidhi Subbaraman, "Science Misinformation Alarms Francis Collins as He Leaves Top NIH Job," *Nature* 600, no. 7889 (December 3, 2021): 372–373, https://doi.org/10 .1038/d41586-021-03611-2.

5. Alondra Nelson, *Body and Soul: The Black Panther Party and the Fight against Medical Discrimination* (Minneapolis: University of Minnesota Press, 2011).

6. Justin Feldman, "A Year In, How Has Biden Done on Pandemic Response?," *Medium* (blog), January 6, 2022, https://jmfeldman.medium.com/a-year-in-how-has -biden-done-on-pandemic-response-88452c696f2.

Epilogue

1. See C. Forsythe and J. Giordano, "On the Need for Neurotechnology in the National Intelligence and Defense Agenda: Scope and Trajectory," 2011, http://www .synesisjournal.com/vol2_no2_t1/Forsythe_Giordano_2011_2_1.pdf; G. K. Gronvall, "US Competitiveness in Synthetic Biology," *Health Security* 13, no. 6 (2015): 378–389, https://doi.org/10.1089/hs.2015.0046.

2. See, e.g., Joel Garreau, *Radical Evolution: The Promise and Peril of Enhancing Our Minds, Our Bodies—and What It Means to Be Human* (New York: Broadway Books, 2005), http://books.google.com/books?id=THGv6naLEu4C&printsec=frontcover&dq =garreau+radical+evolution&hl=&cd=2&source=gbs_api; Nicholas Greig Evans and Michael J. Selgelid, "Biosecurity and Open-Source Biology: The Promise and Peril of Distributed Synthetic Biological Technologies," *Science and Engineering Ethics* 21, no. 4 (September 2014): 1065–1083, https://doi.org/10.1007/s11948-014-9591-3; Robert H. Carlson, *Biology Is Technology: The Promise, Peril, and New Business of Engineering Life* (Cambridge, MA: Harvard University Press, 2010), https://doi.org/10.2307/j.ctt13x0hz9.

But cf. Gigi Gronvall *Synthetic Biology: Safety, Security, and Promise* (Baltimore, MD: Health Security Press, 2016).

3. See, e.g., Maryn McKenna, *Superbug: The Fatal Menace of MRSA* (New York: Free Press, 2010).

4. Nicholas G. Evans, "Dual-Use Decision Making: Relational and Positional Issues," *Monash Bioethics Review* 32, no. 3–4 (2014): 268–283, https://doi.org/10.1007/s40592 -015-0026-y.

5. Schwartz, personal communication, June 2017, Northwestern University.

6. Bipartisan Commission on Biodefense, "The Apollo Program for Biodefense— Winning the Race Against Biological Threats," 2021, https://biodefensecommission .org/reports/the-apollo-program-for-biodefense-winning-the-race-against-biological -threats/.

7. Chris McGreal, "Why Joe Lieberman Is Holding Barack Obama to Ransom over Healthcare," *The Guardian*, December 16, 2009, http://www.theguardian.com/world /2009/dec/16/joe-lieberman-barack-obama-us-healthcare.

8. Rob Copeland, "The Secret Group of Scientists and Billionaires Pushing a Manhattan Project for Covid-19," *Wall Street Journal*, April 27, 2020, sec. US, https:// www.wsj.com/articles/the-secret-group-of-scientists-and-billionaires-pushing-trump -on-a-covid-19-plan-11587998993.

9. Peter Navarro, "Memorandum to the Task Force through COS and NSA" February 9, 2020. https://www.sciencemag.org/sites/default/files/manhattan%20project%20 bright%20exhibit%2021.pdf.

10. Nicholas Greig Evans, Maimuna S. Majumder, and Tara C. Smith, *Ebola's Message: Public Health and Medicine in the 21st Century* (Cambridge, MA: MIT Press, 2016).

11. For the military version of this, see Evans, *The Ethics of Neuroscience and National Security*.

12. Robert Carlson, "Senator Bill Frist's Biological 'Manhattan Project,'" synthesis, accessed January 26, 2021, http://www.synthesis.cc/synthesis/2005/06/senator_bill _frists_biological_manhattan_project.

13. Sharon Weinberger, *The Imagineers of War: The Untold Story of DARPA, the Pentagon Agency That Changed the World* (New York: Vintage, 2017).

14. Robert Carlson and Roger Brent, "DARPA Open Source Biology Letter," synthesis, accessed January 26, 2021, http://www.synthesis.cc/darpa-open-source-biology-letter.

15. Bill Frist, "2005: Frist Calls for Manhattan Project for the 21st Century," Bill Frist: public speaker, former Senate majority leader and cardiothoracic surgeon, July 7, 2020, http://billfrist.com/2005-frist-calls-for-manhattan-project-for-the-21st-century/.

16. Maryn McKenna, "THE PANDEMIC VACCINE PUZZLE Part 7: Time for a Vaccine 'Manhattan Project'?," CIDRAP, accessed January 26, 2021, https://www.cidrap.umn.edu/news-perspective/2007/11/pandemic-vaccine-puzzle-part-7-time-vaccine-manhattan-project.

17. Mark Erikson, *Into the Unknown Together: The DOD, NASA, and Early Spaceflight*, report number ADA459973 (Maxwell AFB: Air University Press, 2005); Diane Vaughan, *The Challenger Launch Decision: Risky Technology, Culture, and Deviance at NASA* (Chicago: University of Chicago Press, 2016); Albert K. Lai, *The Cold War, the Space Race, and the Law of Outer Space: Space for Peace* (Abingdon, UK: Routledge, 2021).

18. Lillian Hoddeson and Gordon Baym, *Critical Assembly: A Technical History of Los Alamos during the Oppenheimer Years, 1943–1945* (Cambridge: Cambridge University Press, 1993), http://lccn.loc.gov/92036611.

19. Peter J. Westwick, "Secret Science: A Classified Community in the National Laboratories," *Minerva* 38, no. 4 (2000): 363–391, https://doi.org/10.1023/A:1004801129528.

20. See, e.g., Jon Else, *The Day after Trinity*, Documentary, Biography (KTEH, 1981).

21. Eileen Welsome, *The Plutonium Files, America's Secret Medical Experiments in the Cold War* (Delta Press, 2000).

22. Gill Scott-Heron, "Whitey on the Moon," *A New Black Poet—Small Talk at 125th and Lenox*, Flying Dutchman/RCA, 1970, 33⅓ rpm.

23. Alex John London and Jonathan Kimmelman, "Against Pandemic Research Exceptionalism," *Science*, April 23, 2020, https://doi.org/10.1126/science.abc1731.

24. Nicholas G. Evans, "Human Infection Challenge Studies: A Test for the Social Value Criterion of Research Ethics," *MSphere* 5, no. 4 (August 26, 2020), https://doi.org/10.1128/mSphere.00669-20.

25. Jerry Avorn and Aaron Kesselheim, "Regulatory Decision-Making on COVID-19 Vaccines during a Public Health Emergency," *JAMA* 324, no. 13 (October 6, 2020): 1284–1285, https://doi.org/10.1001/jama.2020.17101; Sandra Crouse Quinn et al., "Public Willingness to Take a Vaccine or Drug Under Emergency Use Authorization during the 2009 H1N1 Pandemic," *Biosecurity and Bioterrorism: Biodefense Strategy, Practice, and Science* 7, no. 3 (September 1, 2009): 275–290, https://doi.org/10.1089/bsp.2009.0041.

26. "Data Show Panic, Disorganization Dominate the Study of Covid-19 Drugs," *STAT* (blog), July 6, 2020, https://www.statnews.com/2020/07/06/data-show-panic-and-disorganization-dominate-the-study-of-covid-19-drugs/.

27. Matthew Herper, "Inside the NIH's Controversial Decision to Stop Its Big Remdesivir Study," *STAT* (blog), May 11, 2020, https://www.statnews.com/2020/05/11/inside-the-nihs-controversial-decision-to-stop-its-big-remdesivir-study/.

28. Sean McDonald, "Ebola: A Big Data Disaster," accessed December 31, 2020, https://www.academia.edu/21348760/Ebola_A_Big_Data_Disaster.

29. David Hunter and Nicholas Evans, "Facebook Emotional Contagion Experiment Controversy," *Research Ethics* 12, no. 1 (January 1, 2016): 2–3, https://doi.org/10.1177/1747016115626341.

30. Two National Research Council Reports on "dual-use research," in their ultimate recommendations, make strong mention of the role of open and unfettered life sciences in producing both knowledge and technology. See National Research Council, "Biotechnology Research in an Age of Terrorism" (Washington, DC: National Academies Press, February 2004); National Research Council, "Globalization, Biosecurity, and the Future of the Life Sciences" (National Academies Press, 2006).

31. Ryan Muldoon, "Diversity and the Division of Cognitive Labor," *Philosophy Compass* 8, no. 2 (2013): 117–125, https://doi.org/10.1111/phc3.12000; Ryan Muldoon and Michael Weisberg, "Robustness and Idealization in Models of Cognitive Labor," *Synthese* 183, no. 2 (July 2010): 161–174, https://doi.org/10.1007/s11229-010-9757-8.

32. Paul P. Glasziou, Sharon Sanders, and Tammy Hoffmann, "Waste in Covid-19 Research," *BMJ* 369 (May 12, 2020): m1847, https://doi.org/10.1136/bmj.m1847; Paul Elias Alexander et al., "COVID-19 Coronavirus Research Has Overall Low Methodological Quality Thus Far: Case in Point for Chloroquine/Hydroxychloroquine," *Journal of Clinical Epidemiology* 123 (July 1, 2020): 120–126, https://doi.org/10.1016/j.jclinepi.2020.04.016.

33. Daniel P. Oran and Eric J. Topol, "Prevalence of Asymptomatic SARS-CoV-2 Infection," *Annals of Internal Medicine* 173, no. 5 (June 3, 2020): 362–367, https://doi.org/10.7326/M20-3012; Jingjing He et al., "Proportion of Asymptomatic Coronavirus Disease 2019: A Systematic Review and Meta-Analysis," *Journal of Medical Virology* 93, no. 2 (February 2021): 820–830, https://doi.org/10.1002/jmv.26326; Lucy Rivett et al., "Screening of Healthcare Workers for SARS-CoV-2 Highlights the Role of Asymptomatic Carriage in COVID-19 Transmission," ed. Jos WM van der Meer, *ELife* 9 (May 11, 2020): e58728, https://doi.org/10.7554/eLife.58728; Mercedes Yanes-Lane et al., "Proportion of Asymptomatic Infection among COVID-19 Positive Persons and Their Transmission Potential: A Systematic Review and Meta-Analysis," *PLOS ONE* 15, no. 11 (November 3, 2020): e0241536, https://doi.org/10.1371/journal.pone.0241536; Andreas Kronbichler et al., "Asymptomatic Patients as a Source of COVID-19 Infections: A Systematic Review and Meta-Analysis," *International Journal of Infectious Diseases: IJID: Official Publication of the International Society for Infectious Diseases* 98 (September 2020): 180–186, https://doi.org/10.1016/j.ijid.2020.06.052.

34. Helen Branswell and Megan Thielking, "Fluctuating Funding and Flagging Interest Hurt Coronavirus Research," *STAT* (blog), February 10, 2020, https://www.statnews.com/2020/02/10/fluctuating-funding-and-flagging-interest-hurt-coronavirus-research/.

35. Jason L. Schwartz, "The Spanish Flu, Epidemics, and the Turn to Biomedical Responses," *American Journal of Public Health* 108, no. 11 (September 25, 2018): 1455–1458, https://doi.org/10.2105/AJPH.2018.304581.

36. Nicholas B. King, "The Ethics of Biodefense," *Bioethics* 19, no. 4 (2005): 432–446, https://doi.org/10.1111/j.1467-8519.2005.00454.x.

37. T. V. Inglesby, R. Grossman, and T. O'Toole, "A Plague on Your City: Observations from TOPOFF," *Clinical Infectious Diseases: An Official Publication of the Infectious Diseases Society of America* 32, no. 3 (February 1, 2001): 436–445, https://doi.org/10.1086/318513; Tara O'Toole, Mair Michael, and Thomas V. Inglesby, "Shining Light on 'Dark Winter,'" *Clinical Infectious Diseases* 34, no. 7 (April 1, 2002): 972–983, https://doi.org/10.1086/339909.

38. Johns Hopkins Center for Health Security, "PUBLIC-PRIVATE COOPERATION FOR PANDEMIC: PREPAREDNESS AND RESPONSE A CALL TO ACTION," 2019, https://www.centerforhealthsecurity.org/event201/event201-resources/200117-PublicPrivatePandemicCalltoAction.pdf; Johns Hopkins Center for Health Security, "Implications of Clade X for Policy," 2018, https://www.centerforhealthsecurity.org/our-work/events/2018_clade_x_exercise/pdfs/Clade-X-policy-statements.pdf.

39. Johns Hopkins Center for Health Security, "PUBLIC-PRIVATE COOPERATION"; "Implications of Clade X."

40. Donald A. Henderson, Thomas V. Inglesby Jr., Rita Grossman, and Tara O'Toole, "A Plague on Your City: Observations from TOPOFF," *Clinical Infectious Diseases* 32, no. 3 (February 1, 2001): 436–445, https://doi.org/10.1086/318513.

41. Kyle Mizokami, "The U.S. Lost a (Fictional) War with Iran 18 Years Ago," *Popular Mechanics*, January 3, 2020, https://www.popularmechanics.com/military/a30392654/millennium-challenge-qassem-soleimani/.

42. Amy Maxmen and Jeff Tollefson, "Two Decades of Pandemic War Games Failed to Account for Donald Trump," *Nature* 584, no. 7819 (August 4, 2020): 26–29, https://doi.org/10.1038/d41586-020-02277-6.

43. Ronald Klain, "I Have Growing Doubts about These Glitzy Role-Playing Events: They Create an Illusion of Improving Preparedness, but Do They? What ACTUAL Progress Has Been Made since the Clade X Exercise? People/Institutions Should Be Play Acting Less, Engaging Policy Makers More. #event201," Tweet, *@RonaldKlain* (blog), October 18, 2019, https://twitter.com/RonaldKlain/status/1185197319337185280.

44. Julia Lynch, Nicholas Evans, Erin Ice, and Deena Kelly Costa, "Ignoring Nurses: Media Coverage during the COVID-19 Pandemic," *Annals of the American Thoracic Society*, February 12, 2021, https://doi.org/10.1513/AnnalsATS.202010-1293PS.

45. Hugh LaFollette, *In Defense of Gun Control*. In chapter 1, LaFollette defends—again, as a long-time gun owner and hunter—the idea that firearms are explicitly

for taking human lives, and that all other purposes are exaptations to the central evolution of the firearm.

46. C. J. Chivers, *The Gun*, 2011, https://www.simonandschuster.com/books/The -Gun/C-J-Chivers/9780743271738; Robert Fisk, "For Patriotism and Profit: An Interview with Mikhail Kalashnikov," *The Independent*, April 22, 2001.

47. Vannevar Bush, *Science, The Endless Frontier* (Washington, DC: United States Government Printing Office, 1945).

Index

Annas, George, 42–44, 47, 49, 58, 61, 70, 83

Biden, Joseph, 160, 163, 167, 186
Bioterrorism, 8–10, 22, 101, 117
  "Nature as the ultimate," 8
Black Panther Party, 185

Civilian immunity. See Noncombatants
Climate change, 9, 33–35, 64, 84–85, 181
Communicable disease, 13, 20, 74–76, 87–88, 97, 106, 181–183
Contract theories of ethics, 95–99, 109–110

Daszak, Peter, 19–20, 128
Disability, 38, 68, 93–94, 108–109, 126
Discrimination (just war), 53–54, 135, 145–147, 185
Doctrine of double effect, 52
Domestic violence, 6, 38, 142
Domination, 85–88, 140–146

Ebola virus disease, 23–24, 85, 119, 122–123, 194
Effectiveness, 39, 50, 88, 140
Essential personnel, 143, 149, 154–156

Fauci, Anthony, 94, 161, 163

Gostin, Lawrence, 41–44, 47–50, 57–58, 61, 91, 96, 117

Healthcare workers, 30, 80, 139, 143, 153–159
Health security
  definition of, 7–8
  public health and, 57–58
  relation to public health ethics, 10, 39–41
  relation to the state, 92–94
  securitization and, 21–25
HIV/AIDS, 22–25, 42–43, 68, 86, 94, 163, 167
Hobbes, Thomas, 94

Impersonal account of disease. See Threat
Infectious disease
  criminalization of, 49, 64, 71
  distinctiveness, 20
  patient as victim and vector view of, 71–78, 100
  securitization of, 21–28
Influenza, 28–29, 68–69, 107, 110, 139, 192
International health regulations, 7, 10, 22, 25, 134–135
International humanitarian law, 55, 134–136, 157–158
Isolation, 42, 54, 63, 74, 85, 120, 138, 149, 151

Kass, Nancy, 46, 55, 103

Labor, and infectious disease, 102, 107–108, 144, 162, 180

Last resort, 34, 53, 76, 80
Least infringement, 44, 43, 144
Least restrictive means, 41, 44, 145
Legitimate authority, 57, 91–93
Liberal neutrality. See Neutrality
Libertarianism, 47–49, 95–97
Long COVID, 6, 109, 170

Masking, 139, 156, 167, 199, 201
May, Larry, 11, 55, 82, 136
Model State Health Emergency Powers
    Act, 10, 40–44, 117–118
Moehler, Michael, 93, 105, 107, 111

Necessity, 9, 41, 70, 135–137
Neutrality, 178–179
Noncombatants, 34–35, 52, 76, 89, 121,
    131–145

Opioids. See Overdoses
Orthodox view, of public health ethics,
    39–45
Overdoses, 25, 123

Pacificism
    contingent, 81–83, 136
    and just war theory, 45, 61
    and realism, 82, 86
Panic and neglect, 30, 35, 50, 195
Patient as victim and vector, 71–78
Political philosophy, 93–98
Prevention
    In public health, 31, 56
    In public health emergencies, 125
    In war, 124–125
Proportionality, 51–52, 54, 88, 125–127,
    135, 145
Public health emergency
    of international concern (PHEIC), 15,
    23, 84, 116–117
    just cause for, 122–124
Public justification, 54, 147–148

Quarantine, 9, 34, 54, 74, 99, 120, 148

Rationing. See Resource allocation
Reagan, Ronald, 68, 79
Resource allocation, 2, 30, 34,
    100, 156
Rights
    to health, 58, 99, 101
    to security, 145–146
    waiving of, 73

Social distancing, 3, 138–150
State liability, 85, 135–137, 145–147
Surgeon General of the United States,
    28, 30, 160, 163–165
Surveillance, 46, 109, 124, 144

Threat
    impersonal account of disease and,
        78–81
    in public health, 26–29, 49–50, 57,
        66–71, 119, 122, 137
    in war, 51–52, 55, 96, 137
Trump, Donald J., 3–4, 27, 63–64, 163

Unlimited liability thesis, 157
Utilitarianism, 100–102

Vaccines, 6–7, 44, 48, 77, 129,
    133–134, 183

War. See also War on Terror
    on AIDS, 67–68
    as an analogy, 1, 27, 35, 65, 81, 169,
        177, 196
    as a catastrophe, 48, 127
    between states, 53, 70
War on Terror, 20, 25, 60, 64, 92,
    112
World Health Organization, 2, 4,
    115–116, 118, 133
    and health security, 7–8, 23–25